T0263948

Changing Paradigms in Diagnosis and Treatment of Urolithiasis

Guest Editors

CARL A. OSBORNE, DVM, PhD
JODY P. LULICH, DVM, PhD

VETERINARY CLINICS OF NORTH AMERICA: SMALL ANIMAL PRACTICE

www.vetsmall.theclinics.com

January 2009 • Volume 39 • Number 1

SAUNDERS an imprint of ELSEVIER, Inc.

W.B. SAUNDERS COMPANY
A Division of Elsevier Inc.

1600 John F. Kennedy Blvd. ● Suite 1800 ● Philadelphia, PA 19103-2899

http://www.vetsmall.theclinics.com

VETERINARY CLINICS OF NORTH AMERICA: Volume 39, Number 1
SMALL ANIMAL PRACTICE
January 2009 ISSN 0195-5616, ISBN-13: 978-1-4377-0560-7, ISBN-10: 1-4377-0560-X

Editor: John Vassallo; j.vassallo@elsevier.com
Developmental Editor: Theresa Collier

© **2008 Elsevier** ■ **All rights reserved.**

This journal and the individual contributions contained in it are protected under copyright by Elsevier, and the following terms and conditions apply to their use:

Photocopying
Single photocopies of single articles may be made for personal use as allowed by national copyright laws. Permission of the Publisher and payment of a fee is required for all other photocopying, including multiple or systematic copying, copying for advertising or promotional purposes, resale, and all forms of document delivery. Special rates are available for educational institutions that wish to make photocopies for non-profit educational classroom use. For information on how to seek permission visit www.elsevier.com/permissions or call: (+44) 1865 843830 (UK)/(+1) 215 239 3804 (USA).

Derivative Works
Subscribers may reproduce tables of contents or prepare lists of articles including abstracts for internal circulation within their institutions. Permission of the Publisher is required for resale or distribution outside the institution. Permission of the Publisher is required for all other derivative works, including compilations and translations (please consult www.elsevier.com/permissions).

Electronic Storage or Usage
Permission of the Publisher is required to store or use electronically any material contained in this journal, including any article or part of an article (please consult www.elsevier.com/permissions). Except as outlined above, no part of this publication may be reproduced, stored in a retrieval system or transmitted in any form or by any means, electronic, mechanical, photocopying, recording or otherwise, without prior written permission of the Publisher.

Notice
No responsibility is assumed by the Publisher for any injury and/or damage to persons or property as a matter of products liability, negligence or otherwise, or from any use or operation of any methods, products, instructions or ideas contained in the material herein. Because of rapid advances in the medical sciences, in particular, independent verification of diagnoses and drug dosages should be made.

Although all advertising material is expected to conform to ethical (medical) standards, inclusion in this publication does not constitute a guarantee or endorsement of the quality or value of such product or of the claims made of it by its manufacturer.

Veterinary Clinics of North America: Small Animal Practice (ISSN 0195-5616) is published bimonthly (For Post Office use only: volume 39 issue 1 of 6) by Elsevier Inc., 360 Park Avenue South, New York, NY 10010-1710. Months of issue are January, March, May, July, September, and November. Business and Editorial Offices: 1600 John F. Kennedy Blvd., Suite 1800, Philadelphia, PA 19103-2899. Customer Service Office: 11830 Westline Industrial Drive, St. Louis, MO 63146. Periodicals postage paid at New York, NY and additional mailing offices. Subscription prices are $229.00 per year (domestic individuals), $366.00 per year (domestic institutions), $114.00 per year (domestic students/residents), $303.00 per year (Canadian individuals), $450.00 per year (Canadian institutions), $336.00 per year (international individuals), $450.00 per year (international institutions), and $165.00 per year (international and Canadian students/residents). To receive student/resident rate, orders must be accompanied by name of affiliated institution, date of term, and the *signature* of program/residency coordinator on institution letterhead. Orders will be billed at individual rate until proof of status is received. Foreign air speed delivery is included in all *Clinics* subscription prices. All prices are subject to change without notice. **POSTMASTER:** Send address changes to *Veterinary Clinics of North America: Small Animal Practice*, 11830 Westline Industrial Drive, St. Louis, MO 63146. Customer Service (orders, claims, online, change of address): Elsevier Periodicals Customer Service, 11830 Westline Industrial Drive, St. Louis, MO 63146. Tel: 1-800-654-2452 (U.S. and Canada). Fax: 314-523-5170. E-mail: journalscustomerservice-usa@elsevier.com (for print support); journalsonlinesupport-usa@elsevier.com (for online support).

Reprints. For copies of 100 or more of articles in this publication, please contact the Commercial Reprints Department, Elsevier Inc., 360 Park Avenue South, New York, NY 10010-1710. Tel.: 212-633-3812; Fax: 212-462-1935; E-mail: reprints@elsevier.com.

Veterinary Clinics of North America: Small Animal Practice is also published in Japanese by Inter Zoo Publishing Co., Ltd., Aoyama Crystal-Bldg 5F, 3-5-12 Kitaaoyama, Minato-ku, Tokyo 107-0061, Japan.

Veterinary Clinics of North America: Small Animal Practice is covered in *Current Contents/Agriculture, Biology and Environmental Sciences, Science Citation Index, ASCA, MEDLINE/PubMed (Index Medicus), Excerpta Medica,* and *BIOSIS.*

Printed and bound in the United Kingdom
Transferred to Digital Print 2011

Contributors

GUEST EDITORS

CARL A. OSBORNE, DVM, PhD
Diplomate, American College of Veterinary Internal Medicine; Professor, Veterinary Clinical Sciences Department, Minnesota Urolith Center, College of Veterinary Medicine, University of Minnesota, St. Paul, Minnesota

JODY P. LULICH, DVM, PhD
Diplomate, American College of Veterinary Internal Medicine; Professor, Veterinary Clinical Sciences Department, Minnesota Urolith Center, College of Veterinary Medicine, University of Minnesota, St. Paul, Minnesota

AUTHORS

LARRY G. ADAMS, DVM, PhD
Department of Clinical Sciences, School of Veterinary Medicine, Purdue University, West Lafayette, Indiana

HASAN ALBASAN, DVM, MS, PhD
Veterinary Clinical Sciences Department, Minnesota Urolith Center, College of Veterinary Medicine, University of Minnesota, St. Paul, Minnesota

DANIKA BANNASCH, DVM, PhD
Associate Professor, Department of Population Health and Reproduction; Veterinary Medical Teaching Hospital, School of Veterinary Medicine, University of California, Davis, Davis, California

ROSALIE BEHNKE, MS, DVM
Hill's Pet Nutrition, Topeka, Kansas

MICHELLE T. BUETTNER
Veterinary Clinical Sciences Department, Minnesota Urolith Center, College of Veterinary Medicine, University of Minnesota, St. Paul, Minnesota

AMY COKLEY, BS
Veterinary Clinical Sciences Department, Minnesota Urolith Center, College of Veterinary Medicine, University of Minnesota, St. Paul, Minnesota

DRU FORRESTER, DVM, MS
Hill's Pet Nutrition Inc., Topeka, Kansa

DAVID GRANT, DVM, MS
Small Animal Clinical Sciences, Virginia Maryland Veterinary College, Virginia Tech, Blacksburg, Virginia

PAULA S. HENTHORN, PhD
Professor of Medical Genetics, Department of Clinical Studies-Philadelphia, School
of Veterinary Medicine, University of Pennsylvania, Philadelphia, Pennsylvania

LORI A. KOEHLER, CVT
Veterinary Clinical Sciences Department, Minnesota Urolith Center, College of Veterinary
Medicine, University of Minnesota, St. Paul, Minnesota

JOHN M. KRUGER, DVM, PhD
Diplomate, American College of Veterinary Internal Medicine; Department of Small Animal
Clinical Sciences, Michigan State University College of Veterinary Medicine, Veterinary
Teaching Hospital, East Lansing, Michigan

JODY P. LULICH, DVM, PhD
Diplomate, American College of Veterinary Internal Medicine; Professor, Veterinary
Clinical Sciences Department, Minnesota Urolith Center, College of Veterinary Medicine,
University of Minnesota, St. Paul, Minnesota

EUGENE NWAOKORIE, DVM
Minnesota Urolith Center, College of Veterinary Medicine, University of Minnesota,
St. Paul, Minnesota

CARL A. OSBORNE, DVM, PhD
Diplomate, American College of Veterinary Internal Medicine; Professor, Veterinary
Clinical Sciences Department, Minnesota Urolith Center, College of Veterinary Medicine,
University of Minnesota, St. Paul, Minnesota

LINDA SAUER, BS
IT Characterization Facility, University of Minnesota, Minneapolis, Minnesota

GERNOT SCHUBERT, Dr Rer Nat
Urinary Stone Laboratory, Vivantes Klinikum im Friedrichshain, Berlin, Germany

LAURIE L. SWANSON, CVT
Veterinary Clinical Sciences Department, Minnesota Urolith Center, College of Veterinary
Medicine, University of Minnesota, St. Paul, Minnesota

LISA K. ULRICH, CVT
Veterinary Clinical Sciences Department, Minnesota Urolith Center, College of Veterinary
Medicine, University of Minnesota, St. Paul, Minnesota

CARROLL H. WEISS
Director (1991–2002), DCA Study Group on Urinary Stones, Dalmatian Club of America,
Sunrise, Florida

JAMES F. WILSON, DVM, JD
Priority Veterinary Management Consultants, Yardley, Pennsylvania

Contents

THE CLINICS ARE NOW AVAILABLE ONLINE!

Access your subscription at:
www.theclinics.com

Preface

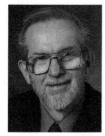 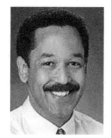

Carl A. Osborne, DVM, PhD   Jody P. Lulich, DVM, PhD
Guest Editors

Our Mission is to enhance the quality and quantity of life of companion animals. We are committed to development of noninvasive methods that will consistently and safely prevent and cure diseases of the urinary system.
   Our Mission encompasses compassionate utilization of contemporary science and selection of clinical teams to provide care that we would select for ourselves. We are dedicated to the welfare of our patients first–and last!

   Mission Statement of the Minnesota Urolith Center, University of Minnesota, Saint Paul, MN

The preface of a symposium on canine urolithiasis published in the March 1986 issue of the *Veterinary Clinics of North America: Small Animal Practice* stated in part:

A nineteenth-century philosopher, Theodor Biroth, penned this thought: 'It is a most gratifying sign of rapid progress of our time that our best textbooks become antiquated so quickly.' It is our hope that the information contained in this issue will rapidly become antiquated as a result of continued research, ultimately leading to the prevention of uroliths.[1]

   Since 1986, our hope became a reality, as evidenced by the growth of knowledge about the causes, consequences, detection, and innovative methods of nonsurgical dissolution and prevention of all forms of canine urolithiasis. The January 1999 issue of the *Veterinary Clinics of North America: Small Animal Practice* (titled "The ROCKet Science of Canine Urolithiasis") provided additional information.[2] As summarized in the article titled "Medical Dissolution and Prevention of Canine Uroliths," "urolithiasis is no longer solely the province of the surgeon."[3]
   The time has passed when feline sterile struvite uroliths require surgery to be removed. Surgical removal of other types of uroliths, notably canine infection-induced struvite, canine cystine, and salts of urate, is moving toward an antiquated status. However, as discussed in several articles in this issue, we still are in search of effective methods to dissolve calcium oxalate, calcium phosphate, and silica uroliths.
   During the past 2 years, we have become aware of a new mineral type of urolith in dogs and cats that consume pet food adulterated with combination of melamine and

Vet Clin Small Anim 39 (2008) xi–xii
doi:10.1016/j.cvsm.2008.10.004
vetsmall.theclinics.com
0195-5616/08/$ – see front matter © 2008 Elsevier Inc. All rights reserved.

cyanuric acid. When cats or dogs consume melamine and cyanuric acid in sufficient quantities, acute renal failure and urolithiasis often occur. Recently, we have learned that human infants who have consumed milk formula adulterated with melamine also form uroliths.

We have made significant progress in our "War on Urolithiasis."[4] With your continued help, we can move ever closer to the day that surgery is no longer needed to remove most uroliths. However, that day has not arrived yet. Keeping this objective in clear focus, please join us in our efforts to hasten the arrival of the day when countless lives will be spared suffering and death from urinary stones. We need your knowledge and wisdom in our efforts to leave "no stone unturned" as we strive to unearth and eliminate the causes of urolithiasis. Cornerstones have been placed, but we are dependent on your help to continue to build the foundation that will result in the development of safe, effective, and practical medical protocols that will consistently dissolve or prevent all types of uroliths.

We thank John Vassallo, editor of this journal, for his nurturing patience. In our experience, this refreshing quality is acquired only by a few editors. They recognize that the quality of an article will be remembered long after the time to compose it is forgotten.

Carl A. Osborne, DVM, PhD

Jody P. Lulich, DVM, PhD
Veterinary Clinical Sciences Department
Minnesota Urolith Center
College of Veterinary Medicine
University of Minnesota
1352 Boyd Avenue
St. Paul, MN 55108, USA

E-mail addresses:
osbor002@umn.edu (C.A. Osborne)
lulic001@umn.edu (J.P. Lulich)

REFERENCES

1. Osborne CA. Foreword: canine urolithiasis II. Vet Clin North Am Small Anim Pract 1986;16(2):209–10.
2. Osborne CA. Preface: the rocket science of canine urolithiasis. Vet Clin North Am Small Anim Pract 1999;29(1):xvii–xviii.
3. Osborne CA. Medical dissolution and prevention of canine uroliths. Seven steps from science to service. Vet Clin North Am Small Anim Pract 1999;29(1):1–15.
4. Osborne CA, Klausner JS. War on canine urolithiasis: problems and solutions. Proceedings of the 45th Annual Meeting of the American Animal Hospital Association, South Bend, IN 1978;569–620.

Dedication

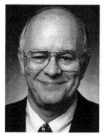

Mark Loren Morris, Jr
February 3, 1934–January 14, 2007

Dr. Mark L. Morris, Jr. earned his Doctor of Veterinary Medicine degree from Cornell University in 1958 and his Doctor of Philosophy degree in nutrition from the University of Wisconsin in 1963. After completing his formal education, he embarked on a career in applied animal nutrition, following the footsteps of his father, Dr. Mark L. Morris, Sr. His mission in life was to focus on the care of animals by nutrition.

Dr. Morris provided insight into the nutritional needs of healthy and ill companion animals (primarily cats and dogs) and so-called exotic and zoo animals. He was admired by colleagues as an innovator, developing the Science Diet brand of premium food and expanding the line of Prescription diets available to complement various recipes of pharmacologic therapy used to treat a variety of diseases. The following tributes are from colleagues and friends.

TRIBUTES

As the president and CEO of Morris Animal Foundation, I had the privilege of working with Mark for more than 3 years. Mark had so many good qualities; he was an animal lover, a scientist, a veterinarian, and a financial wizard who used all of his skills to grow the Foundation started by his parents. Mark was compassionate and caring toward everyone—human and animal. No matter who he was speaking to, he gave that person his complete attention and made sure they knew that what they had to say was important. He loved to be with people.

Mark also tried to make the employees who worked at the foundation feel like they were part of the Morris family. He and his wife, Bette, always welcomed me into their home with open arms whenever I visited Topeka, Kansas. One of my fondest memories was early in my days at the Morris Foundation. We were planning for the foundation's future, and I was feeling stressed. I called Mark. I expressed to him how important it was to me that I preserve his family's legacy and move the foundation in the right direction. He responded, "This isn't my family's foundation. It is your foundation and the staff's foundation. It belongs to all of you."

Over the years, I learned a great deal from Mark, although he never was able to explain hedge-fund investing in a way I could understand! He was a true friend of

Vet Clin Small Anim 39 (2008) xiii–xvi
doi:10.1016/j.cvsm.2008.10.003
0195-5616/08/$ – see front matter
vetsmall.theclinics.com
© 2008 Elsevier Inc. All rights reserved.

mine and a true friend of animals and those that love them. Through his lifetime of work, he touched the lives of millions of animals and humans throughout the world.

Patricia N. Olson, DVM, PhD
President and CEO, Morris Animal Foundation

Mark L. Morris, Jr. was a cherished friend and a wonderful person. He was one of the most caring, intelligent, passionate, enthusiastic, talented, hard working people that I have known. If he were reading these words, he would be appreciative, but also slightly embarrassed. So to save him from that, I will interrupt the accolades with a couple of lighter experiences that will, of course, be at his expense. Here are a few examples of his busy, high-energy approach to daily life. On most topics, Mark was a quick learner, but there were a few exceptions.

Mark was always in a hurry, both at work and the occasional play. As a result of numerous speeding tickets, he was a frequent participant in Kansas' driver safety courses. He probably could have taught the course himself, from memory. While participating in one of the series, he noted to us that his "classmates" were 3 or 4 decades younger than he was and that he was beginning to feel more than a little conspicuous during class. I think he only took one more course after that.

Mark flew a pressurized, turbocharged Beech Baron that had weather radar and wing/prop deicing cuffs. This well-equipped plane, along with his instrument rating, allowed him to fly in questionable weather. This combination caused me, a former fair weather and non-instrument rated pilot, to be in occasional dialogue with the Creator. On one particularly memorable winter night we were returning from California and attempting a landing in Denver, Colorado during a blizzard. We were on the final leg of the approach to the runway, but we couldn't see anything except for snow swirling around the landing lights. Mark was checking his instruments and, at the same time, straining to see the approach lights. I was looking down, through the side window and finally could see the tops of snow-covered trees. In an urgent tone, I advised him that it might be wise to pull up. We climbed slightly and droned on. Thankfully (my perspective), we eventually saw the approach lights ahead and to the right. From there, we landed uneventfully. Mark seemed not to be concerned, and nothing further was said. I reached down and patted the tarmac.

Mark did a great job with presentations we called "wet labs." Attendees were instructed on what to look for when physically evaluating pet foods for quality. It should be no surprise that Mark had a very fast paced, energetic lecturing style. Near the end of the demonstration, he would typically take a bite from a slice of canned Prescription Diet Canine s/d and would quickly chew and swallow it to impress the audience with the quality of the ingredients in the product. For a canned food, s/d was relatively dry. However, he usually took a reasonable sized bite and was able to chew and swallow it in seconds. During one demonstration, in his enthusiasm, he took too large a bite and the chewing went on and on. The attendees, initially amused, soon broke into open laughter. The chewing continued and Mark's face reddened. Finally, he was able to swallow both the food and his pride, and laughed along with us. Then back to his lecture as if nothing had happened.

Now back to the accolades: veterinary medicine, pets, their owners, and the many of us who worked with him owe much to his life's work and the world is not the same without him.

Michael S. Hand, DVM, PhD
Vice-President Emeritus, Hill's Science and Technology Center

Mark Morris was a man of extreme passion. He clearly exhibited this passion through-out his long and distinguished career as it related to the business of therapeutic and wellness diets he and his father developed. While his primary focus was in the area of scientific discovery, he was equally engaged and enthusiastic about all aspects of what was required to deliver a finished product to dogs and cats. Mark's passion spilled over into marketing, sales, manufacturing, quality control, and finance.

Mark was always interested in learning all about people and their individual situa-tions. This usually resulted in long-term personal relationships across virtually all levels of socioeconomic backgrounds. This curiosity not only helped build relationships, but also was a huge benefit in his business activities as well.

Mark gave back to the community in a number of ways. He and I formed the Topeka Zoological Foundation and established the "Lions Pride Exhibit", to cite just one ex-ample. His philanthropy by way of the Morris Animal Foundation is well established.

Robert C. Wheeler
CEO, Hill's Pet Nutrition

I first met Dr. Morris in 1975 when he came to Minnesota to ask for independent stud-ies on the safety and efficacy of a diet that he was formulating. That was the beginning of a life-long relationship. I came to know Mark Jr. as an enthusiastic, cheerful, and generous colleague and friend. His warm smile that he wore inside and out was con-tagious. He was a charismatic person of enormous energy who went the extra mile in his efforts to serve veterinarians by way of application of nutritional principles to clinical veterinary medicine. His training in research combined with common sense and skills in business provided him with unique insights into the needs of colleagues in private practice. In his role as the owner of the research company known as Mark Morris Associates, he surrounded himself with individuals who had expertise in special facets of basic and applied nutrition. Their combined expertise rivaled many clinical nutrition programs in colleges of veterinary medicine. Mark also provided formal nutri-tion courses at colleges of veterinary medicine in North America, especially those that did not have faculty with formal training in veterinary nutrition. Acquisition of new knowledge by veterinarians and veterinary technicians at colleges of veterinary med-icine and veterinary conferences, sponsored by Mark Morris Associates and Hill's Pet Nutrition, helped to change the application of nutrition in veterinary medicine from a cook-book art based largely on empiricism, to a highly sophisticated science built on the foundations of verifiable observations and technology. Currently, veterinary nu-trition impacts every phase of the cause, diagnosis, treatment, and prevention of dis-ease. Because of the nutrition courses initiated by Mark Morris Associates, and carried on to this day by Hill's Pet Nutrition, practitioners today are better able to "First Do No Harm."

During the many years of collaboration between the team at the University of Min-nesota, the team at Mark Morris Associates, and the team at Hill's Science and Tech-nology Center (led by Mike Hand), we, at the University of Minnesota were never asked to sign a confidentiality agreement. We trusted each other to be guided by ethical prin-ciples and moral values. Nor were we ever asked to delay publication of results of our studies in scientific journals until our industrial sponsors first reviewed our findings. There were no discussions or agreements about "trade secrets." The philosophy was consistently to generate and share scientifically accurate information. The atmo-sphere of trust in each other was championed by Mark Jr. The sources of financial sponsorship of research findings published in scientific journals were formally acknowledged.

Ultimately, the win/win relationship created by the University of Minnesota, Mark Morris Associates, and Hill's Pet Nutrition generated scientific knowledge that continues to serve the veterinary profession and the public by providing improved methods to manage urolithiasis and countless other disorders affecting companion animals. In addition, it proved to have direct educational benefits in terms of providing advanced training and financial support for post-graduate veterinarians pursuing residency training and the Master of Science and/or PhD degrees. It provided direct benefits to veterinarians in private practice who were given new knowledge to improve the quality of care they provided for their patients. The relationship also provided a source of revenue for our industrial sponsors, a portion of which was reinvested in additional university graduate training grants and research protocols.

Since the time of Mark's passing, many of his colleagues and friends have stated that he will be remembered as a caring, and compassionate gentleman. Let us pause and reflect what it means to be a gentleman. Webster's Collegiate Dictionary defines a gentleman as, "A courteous gracious man… with a strong sense of honor." Roget's Thesaurus provides the following synonyms for gentleman: well mannered, honorable, refined, and… gentle. Let me paraphrase the thoughts that Joseph A. Mancini wrote in an essay entitled "The Order of the True Gentleman."

The true Gentleman is a man whose conduct proceeds from good will and an acute sense of honesty. His self-control is equal to all emergencies. He does not make the poor man conscious of his poverty, the obscure man of his obscurity, or any man of his inferiority or deformity. The true Gentleman is himself humbled if necessity compels him to humble another. He does not flatter wealth, cringe before power, or boast of his own possessions or achievements. The true Gentleman speaks the truth, but always with sincerity and empathy. His deed follows his word, and he is willing to put the rights and feelings of others before his own. He believes in the concept of serving rather than being served. The true Gentleman is a man with whom honor and virtue are sacred.

I will remember Mark as… a true gentleman.

During his lifetime, it has been my observation that Mark demonstrated generous loyalty to the veterinary profession and his alma mater (Cornell University), steadfast loyalty to Hill's Pet Nutrition, and unconditional loyalty to his friends. He was also extremely loyal to his father, Mark L. Morris, Sr., crediting him with many aspects of the amazing success story that we are all recalling at this time. However, I can say that examination of the evidence indicates that the growth of the Morris Animal Foundation and the Science Diet and Prescription Diet brands were catalyzed by Mark Jr. Mark Sr., who conceived of the concept of prescription diets as an integral component of the management of diseases of animals. Mark Jr. and Bob Wheeler, CEO of Hill's Pet Nutrition, provided the leadership underlying the international reputation of Hill's Pet Nutrition.

Mark's loyalty to me encompassed honesty, trustworthiness, and a passion for scientific inquiry. He stood with me in hard times and good times. Loyalty is the natural response to loyalty, which explains why he touched the hearts of so many individuals, including mine. Having him as a loyal friend was a source of great encouragement to me. I am especially grateful for the opportunity to have worked with him as a colleague. It is indeed a great privilege to be able to call him my loyal friend.

Carl A. Osborne, DVM, PhD

Foreword

*"What we do for ourselves dies with us.
What we do for others lives on."*
— Carl A. Osborne

In 1978, we declared war on urolithiasis. In 1981, we developed the Minnesota Urolith Center to investigate the causes, cures, and prevention of urolithiasis. Using state of the science diagnostic techniques, the Minnesota Urolith Center currently analyzes approximately 55,000 stones per year, which are submitted by veterinarians from 48 countries. Since its inception, the center has analyzed more than 500,000 uroliths from more than 100 species of companion animals (including dogs, cats, rabbits, ferrets, guinea pigs, hamsters, horses, and birds), farm animals (including cows, sheep, goats, and pigs), and wild animals (including elephants, dolphins, whales, hippopotami, kangaroos, mink, monkeys, pandas, snakes, tortoises, turtles, lions, and wolves). With the support of an educational gift from Hill's Pet Nutrition, Inc. and individual donors, we do not collect a monetary fee for this service. Rather, our purpose is to help animals by collecting, evaluating, and sharing epidemiologic data about naturally occurring stone disease and by providing diagnostic information about risk factors to our veterinary colleagues. This type of information cannot be obtained from fee-for-service laboratories. The Minnesota Urolith Center is unique in its ability to obtain data from large populations of animals, thus enhancing discovery of demographic, environmental, and etiologic associations.

We are advocates of the philosophy that the best veterinary teaching hospitals in the world not only use contemporary knowledge; they create it. By studying the epidemiology of urinary stones and then using information about associated risk factors to design studies of the underlying causes of stones, our center pioneered the development of safe, effective, and affordable methods to medically dissolve and prevent sterile struvite, infection-induced struvite, cystine, and ammonium urate uroliths. We currently are studying ways to dissolve and prevent calcium oxalate, calcium phosphate, and silica stones.

We also pioneered the development of nonsurgical techniques to remove uroliths from the lower urinary tract of dogs and cats. These include retrograde urohydropropulsion and voiding hydropropulsion. We recently incorporated laser lithotripsy as a management tool for patients with uroliths that would otherwise require surgery.

With the goal of improving the quality of care that we can collectively provide for our patients, help us rewrite these articles in a future issue of the *Veterinary Clinics of North America: Small Animal Practice* without stating, "The solutions to these stone problems are unknown; further studies are needed." Help us write the article that will symbolize urolithiasis as a historic event at the time of the medical "Stone Age."

Won't you join us in leaving no stone unturned as we strive for this goal? We invite you to submit uroliths to our center for analysis. Consult our website

Vet Clin Small Anim 39 (2008) xvii–xviii
doi:10.1016/j.cvsm.2008.10.002
0195-5616/08/$ – see front matter © 2008 Elsevier Inc. All rights reserved.

(http://www.cvm.umn.edu) for a submission form, follow the link to "Department and Centers" to find the Minnesota Urolith Center, and then follow the menu.

Carl A. Osborne, DVM, PhD

Jody P. Lulich, DVM, PhD
Veterinary Clinical Sciences Department
Minnesota Urolith Center
College of Veterinary Medicine
University of Minnesota
1352 Boyd Avenue
St. Paul, MN 55108, USA

E-mail addresses:
osbor002@umn.edu (C.A. Osborne)
lulic001@umn.edu (J.P. Lulich)

Melamine and Cyanuric Acid-Induced Crystalluria, Uroliths, and Nephrotoxicity in Dogs and Cats

Carl A. Osborne, DVM, PhD[a],*, Jody P. Lulich, DVM, PhD[a], Lisa K. Ulrich, CVT[a],
Lori A. Koehler, CVT[a], Hasan Albasan, DVM, MS, PhD[a], Linda Sauer, BS[b],
Gernot Schubert, Dr Rer Nat[c]

KEYWORDS

- Melamine • Cyanuric acid • Uric acid monohydrate
- Nephrotoxicity • Wheat gluten • Uroliths • Crystalluria

DEFINITIONS
What Is Gluten?

Gluten is a concentrated vegetable protein consisting of a composite of the proteins gliadin and glutenin. These exist, conjoined with starch, in the endosperms of some grass-related grains, notably wheat, rye, and barley. Gliadin and glutenin make up about 80% of the protein contained in wheat seed. Since they are insoluble in water, these proteins can be purified by washing away the associated starch. Worldwide, gluten is an important source of nutritional protein, both in foods prepared directly from sources containing it and as an additive to foods otherwise low in protein.

What Is Rice Protein Concentrate?

Rice protein is a form of concentrated vegetable protein that is made by separating and isolating the protein portion from the carbohydrate portion of rice. It is used in many pet foods as part of the formulation. Rice protein concentrate adds plant proteins that contain little, if any, gluten.

[a] Veterinary Clinical Sciences Department, Minnesota Urolith Center, College of Veterinary Medicine, University of Minnesota, 1352 Boyd Avenue, St. Paul, MN 55108, USA
[b] IT Characterization Facility, University of Minnesota, Minneapolis, MN, USA
[c] Urinary Stone Laboratory, Vivantes Klinikum im Friedrichshain, Berlin, Germany
* Corresponding author.
E-mail address: osbor002@umn.edu (C.A. Osborne).

Vet Clin Small Anim 39 (2008) 1–14
doi:10.1016/j.cvsm.2008.09.010
0195-5616/08/$ – see front matter © 2008 Elsevier Inc. All rights reserved.

What Is Wheat Flour?

Wheat flour is made by grinding cleaned wheat grains. Wheat gluten is the primary protein component of wheat flour. Wheat gluten is made by hydrating wheat flour and mechanically separating the wheat gluten from the starch and other components.

What Is Wheat Gluten?

Wheat gluten is the primary protein component of wheat flour. A vegetable protein, wheat gluten is used as a binding agent to thicken gravy in the manufacture of certain types of pet food.

What Is Melamine?

Melamine is an organic base. Its molecular formula is C3-H6-N6 (**Fig. 1**). It is a small molecule containing a relatively large quantity of nonprotein nitrogen. Melamine-related compounds include cyanuric acid, ammeline, and ammelide (see **Fig. 1**). Although it can be metabolized by some bacteria, it apparently cannot be metabolized by mammals. Melamine is of no known nutrient value to dogs or cats.

Because of its high nitrogen content, melamine has been used as a fertilizer in some parts of the world. It has also been used as an industrial binding agent, a flame retardant, and as a polymer in the manufacture of cooking utensils and plastics (eg, Formica, dishes made of plastic). Addition of melamine and related compounds as ingredients in animal or human food is illegal in the United States. Melamine seems to have a wide margin of safety. If consumed, it is relatively nontoxic to man and animals. In mice and rats, chronic exposure to melamine causes urolithiasis.[1–5] Chronic irritation of the urothelium by uroliths induces urothelial hyperplasia and subsequent urinary bladder neoplasia in these rodents. Melamine has also been reported to cause diuresis in rats and dogs;[6,7] crystalluria in mice, rats, and dogs;[1–3,8–10] and fatal uremia characterized primarily by crystalluria in sheep.[11] Apparently melamine and related compounds do not accumulate in the body. Instead, they are rapidly eliminated by the kidneys.[12] Melamine is a common additive in animal feeds in China. Recently it has been determined that a combination of melamine and cyanuric acid are lethal nephrotoxins in cats and dogs.[13–18] A combination of these two compounds is lithogenic in dogs. The lithogenicity of melamine and cyanuric acid has apparently not been reported in cats; however, these two compounds together have been shown to cause the rapid formation of characteristic microscopic crystals in the urine and renal tubules of dogs and cats.

What Is Cyanuric Acid?

Cyanuric acid is structurally related to melamine (see **Fig. 1**) It is possible that the cyanuric acid in pet food was a result of bacterial metabolism of melamine. It has been used as a stabilizer of chlorine in outdoor swimming pools and hot tubs to minimize the decomposition of hypochlorous acid. Hypochlorous acid tends to lose its potency in sunlight. Cyanuric acid associates with hypochlorous acid and stabilizes its structure but does not affect its antimicrobial potency. Unfortunately, a paucity of data is available about the toxicity of cyanuric acid in mammals. Sodium cyanurate fed chronically to mice and rats caused uroliths, indicating poor solubility.[3]

BACKGROUND

On March 16, 2007, Menu Foods Inc. located in Ontario, Canada, a manufacturer of pet food, issued a voluntary recall of canned pet food because of concerns about adverse effects of some of their products on kidney function of cats and dogs.[19,20] The

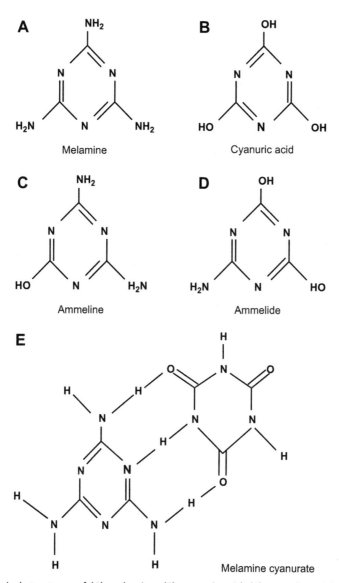

Fig. 1. Chemical structures of (A) melamine, (B) cyanuric acid, (C) ammeline, (D) ammelide, and (E) melamine cyanurate.

recall of pet food was eventually unprecedented in scope, involving an estimated 150 brands manufactured by large reputable pet food companies in addition to Menu Foods. Initially, the food in question was manufactured by Menu Foods between December 3, 2006, and March 6, 2007. On February 22 and 28, 2007, Menu learned about the illness of 2 cats that ate some of their food. At approximately the same date, they received a separate consumer complaint about the death of a cat that ate their food. On March 6 and 7, a company that Menu Foods retained to perform routine tests informed them of the death of one cat and the euthanasia of 2 of 20 other cats in routine palatability studies.[21] On March 9, 4 more cats assigned to the first palatability panel were euthanized because of severe illness. Two cats assigned to a different palatability panel were also euthanized. About the same time, food-related acute to subacute renal failure was diagnosed in dogs and cats in veterinary clinics across the country. Menu Foods contacted the Food and Drug Administration (FDA) on March 15, 2007, and issued a voluntary pet food recall the next day.[21]

Subsequently, on March 23rd, the New York State Food Laboratory reported that they identified aminopterin in samples of food associated with the illness. Initially aminopterin was believed to be the toxin in the recalled pet food. This drug is an antagonist of folic acid that at one time was used to treat cancer. Currently it is used as a rodenticide. The presence of aminopterin was not confirmed by others, however.[16] Testing for other food-related contaminants therefore continued.

Initial tests did not reveal any contaminants in the ingredients. Assays for minerals, heavy metals, ethylene glycol, pesticides, toxins formed by molds, and intentionally added toxins were all negative. Wheat gluten was then investigated as a source of toxins because Menu Foods discovered that production of the problematic food coincided with introduction of wheat gluten from a different supplier in November of 2006. By March 30, melamine was detected in the wheat gluten by Cornell scientists. This observation was confirmed by the FDA.[21] Later it was learned that melamine originating in China was added to wheat gluten. Melamine was also identified in contaminated rice protein concentrate. The FDA then learned that the so-called "wheat gluten" and "rice protein concentrate" were deliberately mislabeled with a code indicating that they were exempt from compulsory inspection by Chinese export authorities because as non-food raw materials they would not be added as ingredients to feeds or food for animal or human consumption. The samples were actually wheat flour and poor-quality rice protein concentrate "spiked" with melamine and melamine-related compounds.[21]

Why would melamine and related compounds be found in pet food? It has been alleged that melamine was added to deceptively increase the apparent protein content of the shipment of wheat flour and rice protein concentrate.[21] How so? The protein concentration of animal and human food is commonly estimated by analysis of total nitrogen content using the Kjeldahl reaction. This method provides only an estimate of the quantity of protein present because it measures both nonprotein and protein nitrogen. In context of melamine, this test would be falsely elevated by the presence of this fake protein. Melamine has a relatively wide safety margin, however. It is unlikely that melamine itself directly caused renal failure in cats or dogs. The FDA later learned that in addition to melamine, cyanuric acid, a substance also containing a relatively high level of nonprotein nitrogen (see **Fig. 1**), and also originating in China, was in the wheat flour, allegedly added with the same deceptive intent.

HOW WAS THE COMBINATION OF MELAMINE AND CYANURIC ACID IMPLICATED?

A significant development in the search for the mystery food-borne toxin occurred when investigators at the University of Guelph's Laboratory Services Division produced a crystalline complex of melamine and cyanuric acid in vitro by adding melamine and cyanuric acid to cat urine.[22] A large quantity of crystals appeared almost immediately. Analysis of the crystals revealed that they were composed of approximately 70% cyanuric acid and 30% melamine and were extremely insoluble. Two other melamine-related substances (ammelide and ammeline) also were identified. Whether these metabolites are also nephrotoxic is currently being evaluated. Additional in vivo studies revealed that melamine alone and cyanuric acid alone were not acutely nephrotoxic. As demonstrated by investigators at the University of Georgia,[13] the University of California,[17] and then at the University of Pennyslvania,[14] the combination of these two industrial chemicals was extremely nephrotoxic, especially to cats. Consumption of melamine and cyanuric acid by cats resulted in extensive lesions in renal tubular epithelial cells associated with numerous characteristic crystals in the renal tubular lumens. The severity of renal dysfunction seemed to be influenced by several factors, including the age of the cat, the quantity of adulterated food consumed, the pH of the stomach and kidneys, and the status of renal health.

FOOD-BORNE OUTBREAKS IN ASIA AND SOUTH AFRICA

The March 2007 pet food–associated renal failure epidemic in North America is similar to a March 2004 epidemic of pet food–associated renal failure that occurred in Asia. In the 2004 Asian epidemic, more than 6000 dogs and cats from Japan, Malaysia, South Korea, Philippines, Singapore, Taiwan, and Thailand were estimated to have developed nephrotoxic renal failure after ingesting a certain brand of manufactured pet food. Compare these data to those from Banfield Hospitals located throughout the United States. Banfield's data were interpreted to suggest that an estimated 39,000 dogs and cats developed renal failure in the 2007 North American food-borne epidemic. A similar food-borne outbreak reported in 2007 in South Africa was attributed to consumption of corn gluten spiked with melamine and cyanuric uric acid.[23]

MINNESOTA UROLITH CENTER INPUT

The Asian epidemic (2004) and the North American epidemic (2007) correspond in many respects to the sudden recognition by our staff of uroliths received beginning in October of 2002 (Fig. 2). These uroliths and crystals were similar (if not identical) in appearance to crystals and uroliths subsequently described by several investigators (Figs. 2–12). The infrared spectrum of the uroliths did not match any of the known minerals in our database. We consulted with several laboratories in the United States; none of them were familiar with the substance in question. We therefore sent representative samples of uroliths to colleagues in Germany for analysis. Samples were evaluated by infrared spectroscopy and solid state nuclear MR spectroscopy; the

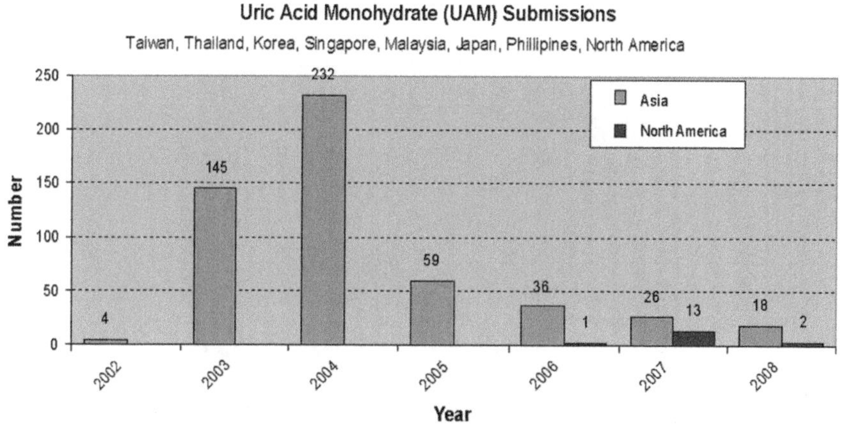

Fig. 2. Number of uroliths containing uric acid monohydrate (or melamine cyanurate?). These uroliths were analyzed at the Minnesota Urolith Center.

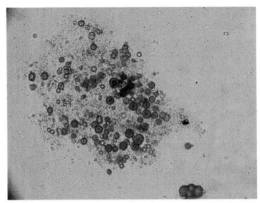

Fig. 3. Photomicrograph of uric acid monohydrate crystals in urine sediment from a dog illustrating unique spherical yellow-brown crystals with radial striations.

analysis revealed findings typical of uric acid monohydrate. This mineral type has recently (2005) been reported in humans.[18] Since 2002, we have received uroliths containing the minerals of interest (uric acid monohydrate or possibly melamine cyanurate) retrieved from 520 dogs and cats living in Asia (see **Fig. 2**). During the period from 2006 to August 11, 2008, we have received 16 uroliths (12 dogs and 4 cats) from the United States containing uric acid monohydrate (or melamine cyanurate).

Staff at the Characterization Facility, University of Minnesota compared our previously unknown samples to references for uric acid monohydrate obtained from the Cambridge Crystallographic Data Center (www.ccdc.cam.ac.uk) using x-ray microdiffraction and electron dispersive spectroscopy. The results were consistent with references for uric acid monohydrate. Comparison of our samples examined by x-ray diffraction and infrared spectroscopy with references for melamine and cyanuric acid did not match. From November 2002 to date, we have been reporting uroliths with these characteristics as uric acid monohydrate (see **Figs. 2–12**).

Greenish-yellow nephroliths were detected in some of the dogs involved in the Asian epidemic (see **Figs. 6, 8,** and **9**). Additionally, crystals were detected in the renal

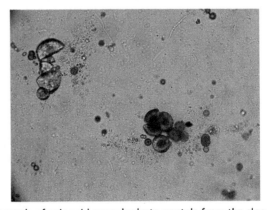

Fig. 4. Photomicrograph of uric acid monohydrate crystals from the dog described in **Fig. 3** illustrating characteristic crystals.

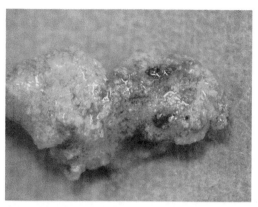

Fig. 5. Photograph of a nephrolith composed of uric acid monohydrate crystals enmeshed in large quantities of matrix. The nephrolith was soft and gooey. This nephrolith was obtained at necropsy from a 13-year-old mixed-breed male neutered dog.

tubules (see **Fig. 6**). The crystals in the kidneys of animals involved in the Asian episode were green-yellow-brown in color, circular in shape, and had striations radiating from their centers. They were identical to the crystals observed in the kidneys of animals involved in the 2007 pet food–associated epidemic and similar (if not identical) to our samples (see **Figs. 3–5**). The Asian endemic of pet food–associated renal failure was attributed to contamination of raw materials with mycotoxins (especially ochratoxin or citrinin) in a pet food manufacturing plant in Thailand. Viewed in retrospect, this diagnosis is unlikely.[24]

ARMED FORCES INSTITUTE OF PATHOLOGY INPUT

Renal tissue from three dogs was submitted to the Armed Forces Institute of Pathology, Washington, DC.[12] Two of the cases were submitted by Idexx Veterinary Services, West Sacramento, California, for light microscopic examination and

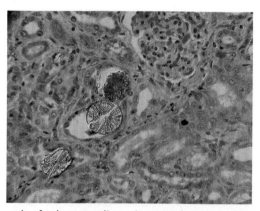

Fig. 6. Photomicrograph of a hematoxylin-eosin–stained section of kidney removed from a 12-year-old mixed-breed dog that had acute renal failure. Note the characteristic appearance of the crystals. The crystals were highly birefringent when examined by polarizing light microscopy.

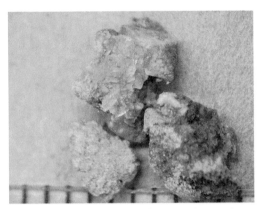

Fig. 7. Photograph of a nephrolith composed of calcium oxalate with prominent surface crystals composed of uric acid monohydrate. This nephrolith was obtained from a 7-year-old male shih tzu.

characterization of the chemical composition of crystals observed previously in hematoxylin and eosin (HE)–stained sections. The third case had been submitted from the Animal Technology Institute Taiwan, Division of Animal Medicine, Chunan, Miaoli, Taiwan, as a Wednesday Slide Conference case submission for the 2004 to 2005 academic year. It was retrieved retrospectively.

Case No. 1 was a 3-year-old female Parson Russell terrier that developed acute renal failure after eating canned food on the Menu Foods recall list. There was no known prior history of renal disease or ethylene glycol exposure. Clinical findings included azotemia and hyperphosphatemia. A complete blood count revealed that neutrophilic leukocytosis was present. Liver enzyme values were within normal limits. The patient died. Necropsy findings included a perforated gastric ulcer, hyperemia and bleeding from the gastric wall, and green crystals in the renal pelves.

Case No. 2 was a 3-year-old spayed female Bernese mountain dog that developed acute renal failure after eating canned food on the Menu Foods recall list. There was no

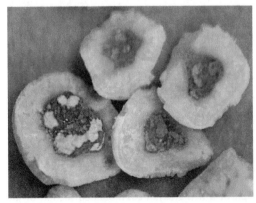

Fig. 8. Photograph of uroliths removed from a dog. Uroliths are composed of an outer layer of magnesium ammonium phosphate (struvite) with an inner core of brown-yellow uric acid monohydrate.

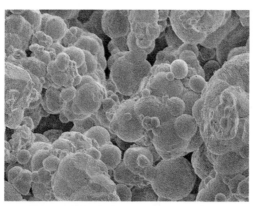

Fig. 9. Scanning electron micrograph of characteristic crystals from the dog described in **Fig. 3**. Original magnification ×500.

known prior history of renal disease or exposure to ethylene glycol. Clinical findings included azotemia, hyperphosphatemia, hyperkalemia, decreased total CO_2, and increased anion gap consistent with acute renal failure and concurrent metabolic acidosis. Because of the severity of the illness, the dog was euthanized. The kidneys were collected at necropsy.

Case No. 3 was a 1-year-old male mixed-breed dog that developed renal failure after eating a commercial dog food for several months. Macroscopic findings included prominent white powderlike deposits in the kidney. Clinical findings neutrophilic leukocytosis and marked azotemia consistent with renal failure.

Light Microscopic Morphology and Histochemistry

In dog No. 1, approximately 90% of the renal tubules were either pale, swollen, and vacuolated, or were occasionally hypereosinophilic and shrunken with nuclear

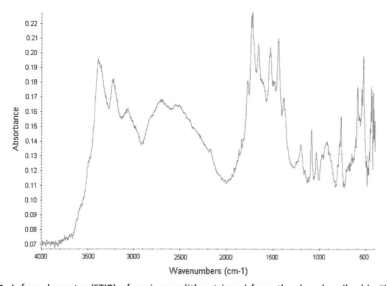

Fig. 10. Infrared spectra (FTIR) of canine urolith retrieved from the dog described in **Fig. 3**.

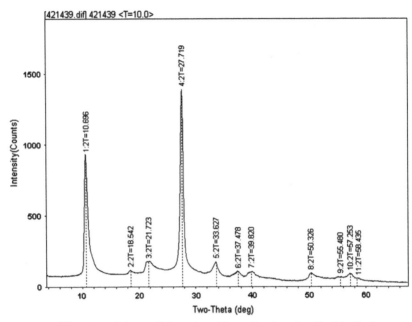

Fig. 11. X-ray diffraction of the urolith retrieved from the dog described in **Fig. 3**.

pyknosis or karyolysis seen on the HE-stained slide samples. The basement membranes of tubules in the inner cortex were thickened and basophilic. There were numerous crystals evenly distributed throughout the cortex and medulla within renal tubules and collecting ducts. The crystals demonstrated bright birefringence when viewed under polarized light. Approximately 75% of the crystals were round, pale brown, and appeared to have a rough surface as a result of smaller crystalline structures being arranged radially and more randomly within the entire birefringent crystal. Some of these crystal structures were arranged in concentric circles. Occasionally, the centers of these concentric circles were empty. The crystals were present within renal tubular epithelial cells and in the lumens of tubules, where they filled and in some areas distended the tubules. The crystals measured up to approximately 80 μm in diameter. Birefringent crystals were also present in the renal pelves. A second type of crystal making up approximately 25% of the birefringent crystals was also present within tubule lumens. Some of these appeared to be in the walls of blood vessels, in addition to the lumens of renal tubules. Low numbers of lymphocytes and plasma cells were observed in the renal interstitium. Similar lesions and crystals were observed on HE-stained sections in dogs No. 2 and 3. Tubular basement membrane mineralization and basophilic nonbirefringent particles were also present in dog No. 3 but were absent in dog No. 2. Similar to dog No. 1, the crystals in dogs No. 2 and 3 were almost exclusively within renal tubules. In dog No. 2, occasional crystals within the renal interstitium elicited a granulomatous inflammatory response with multinucleate giant cells. In dogs No. 2 and 3, the rough pale brown crystals measured up to approximately 100 μm in diameter. There were multifocal aggregates of many lymphocytes, plasma cells, and fewer neutrophils within the interstitium of dog No. 2. Prominent interstitial fibrosis was present in dog No. 3.

In all three cases, Oil Red O72h stain demonstrated variable degrees of the pale brown, rough-textured crystals, indicating a plastic or lipid origin; this stain was

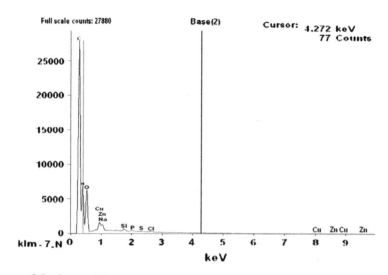

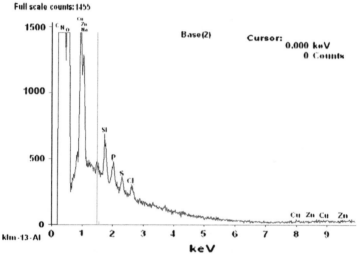

Tue May 29 10:26:04 2007
Filter Fit   Chi-squared value: 365.831
Correction Method: Proza (Phi-Rho-Z)
Acc.Voltage: 15.0 kV Take Off Angle: 35.0 deg

Element	Element Wt.%	Atom %
C	31.54	36.28
N	38.93	38.40
O	29.08	25.12
Si	0.17	0.08
P	0.11	0.05
S	0.08	0.04
Cl	0.09	0.03
Total	100.00	100.00

Fig. 12. Energy dispersive spectroscopy of the urolith retrieved from the dog described in **Fig. 3**.

negative for the smoother platelike crystals. Application of 23 Oil Red O stain for 24 and 48 hours yielded similar results. In dogs No. 1 and 3, Alizarin Red S (pH 4.1–4.3) did not stain either birefringent crystal type. It did stain the basement membranes that were basophilic on the HE sections, however. This finding was consistent with the deposition of a calcium salt other than calcium oxalate, likely calcium phosphate.

The rough, pale brown birefringent crystals demonstrated the infrared spectral characteristics of melamine-containing material. The infrared spectra of the pale brown crystals did not match those of pure melamine or pure cyanuric acid but were similar to spectra obtained at the University of Guelph of a melamine–cyanuric acid complex. Could these be uric acid monohydrate? To produce the same complex, they mixed aqueous solutions of melamine and cyanuric acid in various relative amounts. When the solutions were mixed, spontaneous precipitation of crystals caused the solutions to appear cloudy, but the addition of urea (or formalin) to the solution significantly enhanced the formation of precipitates. The recovered crystals were found to exhibit infrared spectra similar to those obtained from the kidney tissue of the three dogs. The spectra were also the same as those reported at the University of Guelph for urinary crystals from cats and the melamine–cyanuric acid crystals formed in vitro in cat urine.[12]

Scanning Electron Microscopy with Energy Dispersive X-Ray Analysis

Melamine crystals demonstrated peaks for carbon, nitrogen, and oxygen consistent with melamine-containing crystals. The presence of a nitrogen peak in the melamine-containing crystals reflected concentrations of nitrogen in excess of those seen in normal tissue protein.

Scanning electron microscopy with energy dispersive x-ray analysis revealed characteristics of melamine-containing crystals, including a peak for nitrogen, which is not seen when examining tissue protein under normal operating conditions. This finding highlights the high nitrogen content of melamine and, to a lesser extent, cyanuric acid.

Comparison was made of urolith samples submitted from 2002 to date by Asian colleagues, with urolith samples submitted from 2006 to date from United States colleagues. These uroliths were evaluated by x-ray crystallography and electron dispersive spectroscopy. Representative samples from each time period were found to be identical in composition.

Our findings are in agreement with previous reports by Brown and colleagues,[13] Thompson and colleagues,[12] and Cianciolo and colleagues[14] that the pet food-associated renal failure outbreaks in 2004 and 2007 share similar, if not identical, clinical, histologic, and toxicologic findings. We are contacting other colleagues with interest in this phenomenon to resolve the identity of the type of mineral in the uroliths and kidney tissue. Are they uric acid monohydrate, are they metabolites of melamine and cyanuric acid, or are they something else?

NEXT STEPS

It has since been reported that addition of melamine or cyanuric acid to animal feed is a common practice in China. The goal of dishonest exporters is apparently greed because this unethical practice, known as an open secret, is deceptively used to increase the monetary value of poor-quality vegetable proteins (wheat flour, rice protein concentrate, corn gluten, and so forth).

It is beyond the scope of this discussion to provide details regarding when, where, how, and why melamine cyanurate–contaminated food is given to pigs, chickens, fish, ferrets, and humans.[25,26] The cats and dogs that were poisoned with adulterated food may be serving as canaries in the coal mine, however. We are living in a global environment characterized by ever-increasing international trade. This outbreak indicates that our food supply is particularly vulnerable. If such an attack occurred in the face of the strict protocols developed by reputable manufacturers of pet foods, what is the risk that it will happen to human foods? The paradigm change that confronts each of us is to direct our talent, energy, and resources toward a unified effort to "fix the fault" rather than "fixing the blame." More will be accomplished by practicing the thought of "I must do something," rather than that "something must be done."

Because of a generous educational gift from Hill's Pet Nutrition Inc., the Minnesota Urolith Center is able to perform quantitative urolith analysis at no charge. A urolith analysis submission form may be obtained by faxing a request to 612-624-0751 or visiting our Web site, http:www.cvm.umn.edu. Click the link to department and centers to find Minnesota Urolith Center, and click on the icon labeled "How to submit samples."

ACKNOWLEDGMENTS

In addition to the educational gift provided by Hill's Pet Nutrition, parts of this work were performed in the Institute of Technology Characterization Facility, University of Minnesota, which receives partial support from the National Science Foundation through the National Nanotechnology Infrastructure Network program.

REFERENCES

1. Heck HD, Tyl RW. The induction of bladder stones by terephthalic acid, dimethyl terephthalate, and melamine (2,4,6-Triamino-s-triazine) and its relevance to risk assessment. Regul Toxicol Pharmacol 1985;5:294–313.
2. Mast RW, Jeffcoat AR, Sadler BM, et al. Metabolism, disposition and excretion of [^{14}C] melamine in male Fischer 344 rats. Food Chem Toxicol 1983;21:807–10.
3. Melnick RL, Boorman GA, Haseman JK, et al. Urolithiasis and bladder carcinogenicity of melamine in rodents. Toxicol Appl Pharmacol 1984;72:292–303.
4. Ogasawara H, Imaida K, Ishiwata H, et al. Urinary bladder carcinogenesis induced by melamine in F344 male rats: correlation between carcinogenicity and urolith formation. Carcinogenesis 1995;16:2773–7.
5. Okumura M, Hasegawa R, Shirai T, et al. Relationship between calculus formation and carcinogenesis in the urinary bladder of rats administered the non-genotoxic agents, thymine or melamine. Carcinogenesis 1992;13:1043–5.
6. Lipschitz WL, Hadidian Z. Amides, amines, and related compounds as diuretics. J Pharmacol Exp Ther 1944;81:84–94.
7. Lipschitz WL, Stokey E. The mode of action of three new diuretics: melamine, adenine, and formoguanine. J Pharmacol Exp Ther 1945;83:234–49.
8. McPheron T. Pet food contamination found in a new source, rice protein, AVMA advises pet owners to remain vigilant and stay informed [press release] Schaumburg, IL. J Am Vet Med Assoc 2007. Available at: http://www.avma.org/press/releases/070418_petfoodrecall.asp. Accessed November 5, 2008.
9. McPheron T. Melamine and cyanuric acid interaction may play part in illness from recalled pet food [press release] Schaumburg, IL. J Am Vet Med Assoc 2007. Available at www.avma.org/press/releases/070501_petfoodrecall.asp. Accessed November 5, 2008.
10. McPheron T. Fish on U.S. fish farms fed melamine-contaminated feed; FDA discovers contaminated food products from China mislabeled [press release] Schaumberg, IL. J Am Vet Med Assoc 2007. Available at: http://www.avma.org/press/releases/070508_petfoodrecall.asp. Accessed November 5, 2008.

11. Clark R. Melamine crystalluria in sheep. J S Afr Vet Assoc 1966;37:349–51.

12. Thompson ME, Lewin-Smith MR, Kalasinsky VF, et al. Characterization of melamine-containing and calcium oxalate crystals in three dogs with suspected pet food–induced nephrotoxicosis. Vet Pathol 2008;45:417–26.

13. Brown CA, Jeong K, Poppenga RH, et al. Outbreaks of renal failure associated with melamine and cyanuric acid in dogs and cats in 2004 and 2007. J Vet Diagn Invest 2007;19:525–31.

14. Cianciolo RE, Bischoff K, Ebel JG, et al. Clinicopathologic, histologic, and toxicologic findings in 70 cats inadvertently exposed to pet food contaminated with melamine and cyanuric acid. J Am Vet Med Assoc 2008;233:729–37.

15. Dobson RL, Motlagh S, Quijano M, et al. Identification and characterization of toxicity of contaminants of pet food leading to an outbreak of renal toxicity in dogs and cats. Toxicol Sci In press.

16. Maxie G, Hoff B, Martos P, et al. The melamine-cyanuric acid pet food recall. AHL Newsletter 2007;11.

17. Puschner B, Poppenga RH, Loweenstine LJ, et al. Assessment of melamine and cyanuric acid toxicity in cats. J Vet Diagn Invest 2007;19:616–24.

18. Schubert G, Reck G, Jancke H, et al. Uric aid monohydrate-a new urinary calculus phase. Urol Res 2005;33:231–8.

19. Burns K. Recall shines spotlight on pet foods. J Am Vet Med Assoc 2007;230: 1285–6.

20. Burns K, Nolen S, Kahler S, et al. Recall of pet food leaves veterinarians seeking solutions. J Am Vet Med Assoc 2007;230:1128, 1129, 1136–8.

21. Burns K. Witnesses at congressional hearing talk about timing, imports, and surveillance. J Am Vet Med Assoc 2007;230:1601–2.

22. Ruotsalo K. The investigative evolution of the melamine-cyanuric acid pet food recall. Proceedings of the ACVP/ASVCP Annual Meetings, Savannah Georgia, 2007.

23. Anon. Melamine is not a pet food additive. The pet food industry of Southern Africa. Available at: www.petwise.co.za/live/content.php?Item_ID=485. Accessed January 9, 2008.

24. Jeong W, Do SH, Jeong D, et al. Canine renal failure syndrome in three dogs. J Vet Sci 2006;7:299–301.

25. US FDA, Center for Veterinary Medicine. Pet food recall/contaminated feed. Frequently asked questions. 2007. Available at: www.fda.gov/cvm/MenuFpodRecallFAQ.htm. Accessed August 27, 2008.

26. US FDA, Center for Food Safety and Applied Nutrition. Interim melamine and analogues safety/risk assessment. May 2007 Available at: www.cfsan.fda.gov/~dms/melamra.html Accessed August 27, 2008.

Changing Paradigms of Feline Idiopathic Cystitis

John M. Kruger, DVM, PhD[a],*, Carl A. Osborne, DVM, PhD[b],
Jody P. Lulich, DVM, PhD[b]

KEYWORDS

- Feline • Idiopathic cystitis • Lower urinary tract disease
- Pathogenesis

Disorders of the feline lower urinary tract that are characterized by periuria (urination in inappropriate locations), hematuria, dysuria, pollakiuria, and/or urinary obstruction are common but incompletely understood problems. Research over the past 50 years has reaffirmed the notion that cats are similar to other species, including dogs and humans with regard to the fact that lower urinary tract signs may result from a variety of diverse disorders including: bacterial, fungal, and parasitic urinary tract infections; different types of uroliths and urethral plugs; neoplasia, congenital or acquired anatomic or morphologic abnormalities; and traumatic, neurogenic, or iatrogenic causes.[1–4] However, these same studies also serve to emphasize that some young to middle-aged cats are uniquely predisposed to lower urinary tract signs for which precise causes have not be identified. These cats are classified as having idiopathic lower urinary tract disease or idiopathic cystitis. The disorder is believed to affect one quarter to one half a million cats in the United States annually.[5] As of yet, there is no consistent specific diagnostic marker and there is no consistently effective method of therapy.[6]

The term "paradigm" refers to a generally accepted theoretical model that explains complex ideas.[7] Over that past several decades, the prevailing paradigms regarding the causes of cystitis have changed because of: the influence of contemporary studies of the biological behavior of naturally occurring idiopathic cystitis; laboratory models of experimentally induced lower urinary tract diseases; and extrapolation from studies in other species.[8] It is clear, however, that no single model explains all the biological variability observed in cats with idiopathic cystitis. In many respects, feline idiopathic cystitis is a conundrum analogous to an idiopathic lower urinary tract disorder of humans called interstitial cystitis.[9] The extent to which these two conditions share

[a] Department of Small Animal Clinical Sciences, Michigan State University College of Veterinary Medicine, Room D208, Veterinary Teaching Hospital, East Lansing, MI 48824-1314, USA
[b] Veterinary Clinical Sciences Department, Minnesota Urolith Center, College of Veterinary Medicine, University of Minnesota, 1352 Boyd Avenue, St. Paul, MN 55108, USA
* Corresponding author.
E-mail address: kruger@cvm.msu.edu (J.M. Kruger).

Vet Clin Small Anim 39 (2008) 15–40
doi:10.1016/j.cvsm.2008.09.008
0195-5616/08/$ – see front matter © 2008 Elsevier Inc. All rights reserved.

etiopathogenic mechanisms has not yet been precisely defined; however, the diversity in their biological behavior and responses to therapeutic interventions, and their association with comorbid conditions, suggest that these disorders may represent syndromes resulting from a variety of separate underlying but potentially interrelated mechanisms rather than one disease with a single uniform pathogenesis.[8,10,11] Design of effective therapeutic and prevention strategies is ultimately dependent on identifying the specific etiologic factors responsible for feline idiopathic cystitis.

BIOLOGICAL BEHAVIOR

Periuria, pollakiuria, stranguria, and gross hematuria are the most common clinical signs observed in cats with nonobstructive idiopathic cystitis and may precede the obstructive form of the disorder. Remarkably, these clinical signs subside within 5–7 days without therapy in up to 92% of cats with acute nonobstructive idiopathic cystitis.[12–15] Signs may recur after variable periods of time and again subside without treatment. However, recurrences of signs have been reported to affect 39% to 65% of cats with acute idiopathic cystitis within one to two years after the initial episode.[12,14,16,17] In one study, survival analysis revealed that an increased number of prior episodes of lower urinary tract signs was associated with a significantly higher risk of recurrence of clinical signs, while increased age was associated with a significantly lower risk of recurrence of clinical signs.[14] After controlling for age, number of prior episodes of lower urinary tract signs, and diet moisture content, the relative risk that an affected cat will have a recurrent episode of lower urinary tract signs in a 2-year period was approximately 65%. These data and our clinical observations suggest that recurrent episodes of acute idiopathic cystitis decrease in frequency and severity as the cats become older.[13,14,18] Though recurrent clinical signs in patients with idiopathic cystitis are often assumed to be a recurrent episode of the original disease, recurrent signs may also be the result of a delayed manifestation of the original disease (for example, spontaneous or iatrogenic urethral stricture), or a different lower urinary tract disease associated with similar clinical signs (such as urolithiasis).

The authors of this article and others have also encountered a small subset of cats with idiopathic cystitis in which clinical signs persist for weeks to months or which are frequently recurrent.[5,19,20] These cats are classified as having chronic idiopathic cystitis. In the authors' experience, less than 15% of cats that initially presented with acute idiopathic cystitis develop this form of the disease. (Kruger JM, unpublished data, 2003) It has also been the authors' experience that some cats with chronic or frequently recurrent forms of idiopathic cystitis experience spontaneous remission of their clinical signs. Whether chronic idiopathic cystitis represents one extreme in the spectrum of clinical manifestations associated with similar etiologic factors, or whether it represents an entirely different mechanism of disease than that associated with acute self-limiting idiopathic disease is as yet unknown. To date, it appears that the vast majority of studies investigating potential causes of idiopathic cystitis involved cats affected with chronic forms of the disease.

BACTERIAL UROPATHOGEN PARADIGM

In the 1960s and 1970s, the prevailing theory of the cause of lower urinary tract signs was bacterial urinary tract infection (UTI).[21–23] Before 1970, bacterial UTI was one of the most commonly recognized and treated disorders on the lower urinary tract in dogs.[24] Because of the paucity of reproducible evidence about naturally occurring diseases in cats at that time, it was common to extrapolate and apply information derived in other species to cats. The notion that bacteria were commonly involved in feline lower urinary tract diseases was reinforced by erroneous identification and interpretation of bacterial-look-alikes (aka pseudobacteria) found in urine sediment as bacterial pathogens. In a recent study in the authors' laboratory, up to 40% of unstained feline urine sediments classified as positive for bacteriuria by light microscopy were found to be false positives when compared with results of quantitative culture of urine for bacteria.[25] Microscopic examination of unstained urine sediment was associated with only an 11% positive predictive value (ie, the proportion of cats with a positive test that had confirmed bacterial UTI). Staining of urine sediment with a modified Wright-stain procedure (Diff Quik®) reduced the frequency of false positives to approximately 2%.[25,26]

In addition to reliance on faulty results of urinalysis, false-positive bacterial culture results associated with improper urine collection techniques and failure to quantify the number of bacterial isolates were pervasive. As a result, bacterial contaminants were misidentified as bacterial pathogens. The interpretation that bacteria were an important cause of lower urinary tract signs in cats was further enhanced by the observation that clinical signs often subsided in association with antimicrobic therapy. Based on the observation that urinary host defense mechanisms in cats are of such design that cats are innately resistant to bacterial infections,[27,28] it is certain that many affected cats with presumed bacterial UTI appeared to respond favorably to antimicrobics because they had self-limiting forms of idiopathic cystitis.

Although it has been well established that aerobic bacteria account for only 1–3% of bacterial UTI in young to middle-aged cats, empirically selected antimicrobics remain as the most common form of therapy prescribed for cats with hematuria, dysuria, pollakiuria, and periuria.[1–4,28–31] Even though the uselessness of antimicrobial agents in the treatment of abacteriuric cats with lower urinary tract disease also has been well documented, the bacterial UTI paradigm persists.[12]

VIRAL UROPATHOGEN PARADIGM

One attractive hypothesis advanced in the late 1960s and early 1970s implicated viruses as causative agents in the etiopathogenesis of some forms of naturally occurring feline lower urinary tract diseases.[31–33] This hypothesis was supported by the isolation of a gamma herpesvirus (aka bovine herpesvirus type 4), retroviruses (feline foamy virus [FFV]), and a calicivirus (feline calicivirus [FCV]) from urine and tissues obtained from cats affected with lower urinary tract disease.[34–38] Similarly, a number of viral agents including adenoviruses, polyomaviruses, herpesviruses, influenza A, and human immunodeficiency virus, have been associated with hemorrhagic cystitis and other lower urinary tract symptoms in humans.[39,40]

Feline Calicvivirus

The first indirect evidence supporting the hypothesis of a viral etiology in feline lower urinary tract disorders was reported in 1969. Investigators at Cornell University produced urethral obstruction in male cats by urinary bladder inoculation with centrifuged bacteriologically sterile urine obtained from male cats with naturally occurring urethral obstruction.[41] Subsequent isolation of FCV from a Manx cat with spontaneous urethral obstruction, and induction of obstructive uropathy in conventionally reared cats by urinary bladder inoculation with this virus, supported the concept of a viral etiology for feline lower urinary tract disease.[41,42] In a study of induced FCV urinary tract infection in conventionally reared cats, 80% of cats developed urethral obstruction following urinary bladder, aerosol, or contact exposure.[42] However, failure to reisolate FCV from urine after the fourth day of inoculation, lack of a significant serum neutralizing antibody response, and isolation of an additional virus (feline foamy virus) from all obstructed experimental cats, prompted the Cornell investigators to hypothesize that FCV was not a primary causative agent.[32] The notion was advanced that this virus incited other latent viruses present in the urinary tract to induce urethral obstruction. Results of a subsequent study comparing the affects of induced urinary tract infections with FCV alone or in combination with a gamma herpesvirus appeared to support the concept that FCV exacerbated the severity of disease in cats infected with gamma herpesvirus.[31,32]

The questionable nature of the etiologic role of FCV followed reports of other investigators who were unable to obtain reproducible evidence that caliciviruses were associated with naturally occurring lower urinary tract diseases of cats.[3,29,33,36,37] In retrospect, however, inability of investigators to detect FCV in cats with lower urinary tract disorders in the 1970s must be viewed with caution. Their inability to detect FCV appeared to be confounded by improper selection of cases (ie, improper inclusion and exclusion criteria were used to select cats for study), the innately virucidal nature of feline urine, and use of insensitive or inappropriate virus detection methods.[33,43,44] The point to keep in mind is that absence of evidence cannot always be interpreted as evidence of absence.

Feline Foamy (Syncytium-Forming) Virus

Shortly after the isolation of FCV, the Cornell group isolated the syncytium-forming retrovirus FFV (aka feline syncytium-forming virus) from several cats with lower urinary tract signs.[35,36,38] Unfortunately, there are have been limited studies designed to investigate the etiopathogenic role of FFV in cats with lower urinary tract disease.[33] In one study, FCV-induced urethral obstruction in conventionally reared cats was consistently associated with isolation of FFV.[42] In other studies, lower urinary tract clinical signs were not observed in a small number of cats following intravenous, intraperitoneal, intramuscular, intra-articular, or subcutaneous inoculation of FFV.[45–48]

In contrast to other viruses, FFV has been isolated from urine, urinary-tract tissues, and other tissues obtained from a large number of cats with lower urinary tract disease.[33–38] Additionally, FFV antibodies have been detected in serum samples obtained from cats with naturally occurring lower urinary tract disease.[33,38] FFV antibodies have also been detected in a large number of clinically normal cats.[48] The relative ease and frequency with which FFV has been isolated from cats with lower urinary tract signs and the prevalence of FFV antibodies suggests that they may play a potential role in the pathogenesis of the disease. However, it is difficult to assess the relative importance of FFV on the basis of available experimental and clinical evidence. Further investigations are necessary to determine the role (if any) of FFV virus in feline idiopathic cystitis.

Gamma Herpesvirus

In addition to FCV and FFV, investigators at Cornell University isolated a gamma herpesvirus (aka bovine herpesvirus type 4 [BHV-4]) from pooled kidney organ explants obtained from a litter of normal kittens, a kitten with upper respiratory disease, and a kitten with concurrent upper respiratory disease and urethral obstructions.[35,49] Results of studies designed to induce urethral obstruction in specific-pathogen-free (SPF) cats by urinary bladder inoculation of FCV alone, herpesvirus alone, or herpesvirus in combination with FCV, led to the hypothesis that gamma herpesvirus was a primary causative agent in the etiopathogenesis of naturally occurring feline lower urinary tract diseases.[31,32]

In an effort to substantiate Cornell's studies and to further characterize the clinicopathologic manifestations of gamma herpesvirus-induced lower urinary tract disease, the authors inoculated the feline isolate of BHV-4 into the urinary bladders of SPF male and female cats.[50] Results of these studies indicated that BHV-4 was capable of establishing persistent low-grade or latent urinary tract infections in male and female SPF cats. However, in contrast to previous studies, lower urinary tract signs were uncommonly associated with persistent herpes virus urinary tract infections.

Serologic methods also have been used to evaluate the role of gamma herpes virus in feline lower urinary tract disorders. In a prospective study, sera obtained from 167 normal cats and cats with obstructive or nonobstructive idiopathic cystitis, urolithiasis, or bacterial UTI, were evaluated for BHV-4 using an indirect fluorescent antibody test.[3] Antibodies against BHV-4 were detected in sera obtained from 31% of cats with lower urinary tract diseases, and from 23% of normal control cats. However, positive BHV-4 antibody titers were not associated with clinical signs or abnormal laboratory findings. These observations and the inability of other investigators to isolate gamma herpes viruses from cats with naturally occurring lower urinary tract disorders or to induce lower urinary tract signs in healthy cats precludes assigning BHV-4 a primary role in feline idiopathic cystitis. Considering the relatively high prevalence of BHV-4 anti-bodies in the general feline population, additional studies defining the pathogenic role of gamma herpesvirus infections of cats are warranted.[51]

VESICOURACHAL DIVERTICULUM PARADIGM

In the late 1970s and early 1980s, vesicourachal diverticula were cited as playing an etiopathogenic role in cats with lower urinary tract signs.[52,53] A vesicourachal diverticulum is a common congenital anomaly of the urinary bladder that occurs when the portion of the urachus (ie, a fetal conduit that allows passage of urine from the bladder to the placenta during development of the fetus) located at the bladder vertex does not completely close.[54] The result is a blind diverticulum of variable size located in the bladder vertex. Congenital microscopic diverticula are remnant urachal canals lined with urothelium that may persist from the level of the submucosa to the serosa.[55] In a study of 80 feline urinary bladders, microscopic urachal diverticula were detected in more than 40%.[53] Microscopic remnants persisting in the urinary bladder vertex after birth are clinically silent.

Acquired macroscopic diverticula may develop at the bladder vertex of cats with microscopic urachal remnants as sequelae to concurrent but unrelated acquired lower urinary tract diseases (eg, bacterial infections, urolithiasis, crystalline-matrix urethral plugs, idiopathic disease, etc.).[56] Presumably, urethral obstruction and/or detrusor hyperactivity induced by inflammation result in increased intraluminal pressure and subsequent enlargement of microscopic diverticula.[55] Congenital macroscopic diverticula are most likely caused by impaired urine outflow. They develop before or soon after birth and, unlike most acquired diverticula that spontaneously regress, congenital macroscopic diverticula persist indefinitely.

In the early 1990s, many surgeons recommended treatment of vesicourachal diverticula by surgical extirpation.[57,58] The observation that clinical signs coincidentally subsided after diverticulectomy and a lack of studies of the biological behavior of macroscopic diverticula without surgery reinforced the opinion that diverticulectomy was an effective surgical method to eliminate lower urinary tract signs associated with this disorder. Contrary to the prevailing opinion of the time, however, results of clinical studies revealed that diverticulectomy was not required in most cats because adult-onset acquired macroscopic vesicourachal diverticula typically resolved within 2 to 3 weeks after amelioration of clinical signs of lower tract disease.[56] After being resolved, vesicourachal diverticula did not recur in association with subsequent episodes of lower urinary tract disease. These observations provide convincing evidence that most vesicourachal diverticula associated with clinical signs are the result and not the cause of idiopathic cystitis.

STRUVITE CRYSTALLURIA PARADIGM

In the early 1970s, the association between dry diets and lower urinary tract signs in cats became a topic of intense discussion. Also in the early 1970s and continuing for the next decade, several groups of investigators experimentally produced magnesium hydrogen phosphate and then magnesium ammonium phosphate uroliths in normal cats by addition of various types of magnesium salts to their diets.[59] The cats developed typical signs of lower urinary tract disease including urethral obstruction. However, this model did not result in production of struvite-matrix urethral plugs commonly encountered in cats with naturally occurring urethral obstruction.[60] Nonetheless, as the viral paradigm lost popularity in the late 1970s, the general consensus of many investigators and clinicians was that consumption of dry diets with excessive magnesium was an important primary cause of feline lower urinary tract disease.[8]

Beginning in 1983, reports from the Minnesota Urolith Center of medical dissolution of naturally occurring sterile struvite urocystoliths with modified diets corroborated the importance of dietary risk and protective factors in the etiology of sterile struvite urolithiasis.[61,62] In 1985, investigators at the University of California performed studies in normal cats using diets containing alkalinizing and acidifying salts of magnesium.[63] Results of these studies shifted the focus of attention from dietary magnesium to alkaline urine pH as a primary factor involved in the development of struvite crystalluria. Results of these diet-related studies also supported the paradigm in that era that many cases of feline lower urinary tract disease were caused by struvite uroliths and urethral plugs. The pet food industry responded to these recommendations by placing increased emphasis on development of urine acidifying diets modified to dissolve and prevent struvite crystalluria. Many adult feline maintenance diets were modified to minimize struvite crystalluria.[64]

There is abundant evidence that, in past years, sterile struvite uroliths and struvite urethral plugs played a prominent causative role in a substantial number of cats with naturally occurring obstructive and nonobstructive lower urinary tract disease. In addition, dietary factors contributed both to the cause and the treatment and prevention of struvite related lower urinary tract diseases. As a result of dietary modifications by numerous pet food manufacturers in the mid-1980s, the prevalence of struvite uroliths and struvite urethral plugs began to decline (**Fig. 1**). Although struvite continued to be the primary component in urethral plugs (**Fig. 2**), the frequency with which they formed dramatically declined as evidenced by a parallel decline in the number of perineal urethrostomies performed to minimize recurrent urethral obstruction.[65] Unexpectedly, the decline in struvite related urolithiasis was associated with a concomitant rise in calcium oxalate urolithiasis, while, unexplainably, struvite remained as the primary component of urethral plugs (see **Figs. 1** and **2**).

Did the results of these extensive investigations resolve the search for the primary causes of lower urinary tract disease? The observation that signs of hematuria and dysuria occurred in more than 50% of cats with idiopathic cystitis in the absence of any type of crystalluria indicated that other as yet unidentified etiologic factors were also involved.[1–3,14,18]

DYSFUNCTIONAL UROTHELIAL BARRIER PARADIGM

Over the past two decades, urothelial barrier dysfunction has been a pervasive paradigm of causation of human interstitial cystitis.[10,66,67] Likewise, feline studies in the

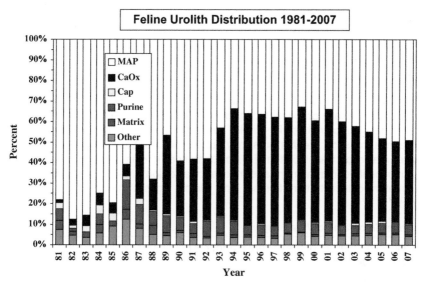

Fig.1. Changing trends in mineral composition of feline uroliths submitted to the Minnesota Urolith Center from 1981 to 2007.

mid- to late-1990s supported the concept that urothelial barrier failure may be involved in the pathogenesis of idiopathic cystitis.[68–70] Bladder urothelium is an important host defense mechanism because it serves as a barrier that prevents entry of uropathogens into deeper structures. Urothelium also selectively controls passage

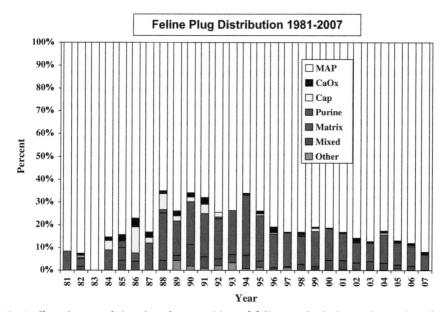

Fig. 2. Changing trends in mineral composition of feline urethral plugs submitted to the Minnesota Urolith Center from 1981 to 2007.

of water, ions, macromolecules, and other solutes across the mucosal surface into underlying tissues.[66,71] Urothelial barrier function largely depends on: 1) specialized high-resistance tight junctions between apical membranes of adjacent urothelial cells; 2) the unique lipid and protein composition of urothelial cell membranes; and 3) a layer of glycosaminoglycans (GAG) located on the luminal surface of urothelial cells.[71,72] There is disagreement as to the relative contributions of the GAG layer and urothelium as the barrier to urine ions, macromolecules, toxins, and microorganisms.[66,72] Regardless, any disease process that: 1) directly injures urothelium; 2) alters structural or functional characteristics of urothelial GAGs or apical tight junctions; and/or 3) disrupts active transport mechanisms may result in loss of barrier function.[72–74] These changes may allow translocation of toxic substances into underlying tissues, resulting in submucosal edema, hemorrhage, neovascularization, mastocytosis, mononuclear inflammatory cell infiltration, fibrosis, and clinical signs of frequency, urgency, and pain.[70,73,75–80]

Defective Glycosaminoglycan Layer

Transitional epithelium of the urinary bladder is covered by a glycocalyx composed of hydrated glycoconjugates, including glycoproteins and glycosaminoglycans (GAGs).[66] Urothelial GAGs minimize adherence of microorganisms and crystals to the bladder urothelium and also limit movement of urine proteins and other ionic and nonionic solutes from the bladder lumen into surrounding tissues.[66,67,81] Quantitative or qualitative defects in surface GAGs and subsequent increased urothelial permeability have been hypothesized to be a causative factor in the pathogenesis of feline idiopathic cystitis and human interstitial cystitis.[20,67,81,82] Chronic exposure of bladder wall tissues to urine constituents could result in sensory afferent nerve stimulation, mast cell activation, and/or induction of immune-mediated or neurogenic inflammatory responses.[10] Compared to normal cats, some cats with idiopathic cystitis appear to have increased urinary bladder permeability to salicylates, urea, and fluorescein, decreased surface GAG expression, and decreased total urinary GAG excretion.[68–70,83,84] Investigators have identified similar abnormalities in humans with interstitial cystitis.[81,85,86] However, others have failed to detect altered urothelial GAG layers, decreased urine GAG excretion, or enhanced urothelial permeability in humans with interstitial cystitis.[87–90] The controversy surrounding the role of GAGs in humans with interstitial cystitis has been confounded by the fact that increased urothelial permeability has been associated with other non-interstitial cystitis lower urinary tract disorders (eg, urolithiasis, chemical cystitis, and bladder overdistention).[10,91,92] Nevertheless, replacement of the urothelial GAG layer with oral or intravesicular administration of pentosan polysulfate sodium (an exogenous semisynthetic GAG analog) appears to significantly reduce the severity of symptoms in some human patients with interstitial cystitis.[93–95] In cats with idiopathic cystitis, however, results of a randomized placebo-controlled clinical trial of oral glucosamine (a GAG precursor) did not reveal any significant difference between the severity of clinical signs in cats treated with glucosamine and those treated with a placebo.[16] Further characterization of structural or functional alterations of the urothelial GAG layer in cats with and without idiopathic cystitis are essential to determine whether these abnormalities are a specific cause of idiopathic disease or a nonspecific effect occurring secondary to other etiologic mechanisms.

Defective Urothelial Proliferation or Differentiation

Urothelium is stratified and consists of at least three layers: a basal cell layer attached to the basement membrane; an intermediate cell layer; and a superficial apical layer composed of large hexagonal cells (so-called "umbrella cells").[71,72] The two deeper layers of urothelial cells serve as progenitors for the overlaying superficial layer. Superficial urothelial cells are responsible for maintaining the bladder permeability barrier and possess unique features including: 1) specialized apical membrane proteins (called uroplakins); 2) high resistance tight junctions between cells; and 3) an active trafficking mechanism designed to insert cytoplasmic vesicles into the apical membrane to accommodate bladder filling.[72] Primary responses of urothelium to injury are desquamation (exfoliation of viable cells), necrosis, and/or apoptosis.[74,96,97] In healthy animals, rapid replacement of exfoliated or injured superficial cells and restoration of urothelial tight junction integrity prevents long-term urothelial barrier malfunction.[98] However, urothelial injury in the face of any disease process that alters normal urothelial proliferation and differentiation could profoundly affect urothelial barrier function.

Urothelial ulceration, tearing, and thinning are common abnormalities identified in biopsy specimens from humans with interstitial cystitis.[99–101] These observations led investigators to hypothesize that impaired urothelial proliferation may be involved in the pathogenesis of human interstitial cystitis.[102] Subsequent identification of abnormal expression of protein biomarkers associated with urothelial growth and differentiation (eg, uroplakins, E-cadherin, ZO-1, glycoproteins, GAGs, and keratins) in biopsy specimens from humans with interstitial cystitis further supported this hypotheses.[66,101,103–105] Also, a novel low molecular weight sialoglycopeptide called antiproliferative factor (APF), which inhibited proliferation of normal bladder urothelial cells in vitro, was identified in the urine of humans with interstitial cystitis.[106] Subsequent in vitro studies revealed that APF suppressed urothelial cell proliferation, increased transcellular permeability, inhibited tight junction protein expression, and reduced growth factor production.[107–109] Unfortunately, detection of urine APF activity as a marker of interstitial cystitis is dependent on bioassays using human urothelial cell cultures. There are no available commercial assays for detection of APF in human or feline urine at this time.[106]

Urothelial ulceration, erosion, and thinning are common light microscopic features of chronic forms of feline idiopathic cystitis.[70,77,80] Despite histopathologic similarities to human interstitial cystitis, there have been relatively few studies evaluating protein biomarkers of urothelial growth and urothelial differentiation in cats with acute or chronic idiopathic cystitis. In a study of three cats with chronic idiopathic cystitis, urothelial cells underlying areas of mucosal erosion expressed abundant levels of the superficial urothelial cell differentiation marker AE-31.[70] However, distribution of AE-31 antigen was altered with staining localized to the perinuclear region of cells rather than at its normal apical membrane position. Likewise, results of a study of 40 cats with chronic idiopathic cystitis revealed that the magnitude of immuno-histochemical staining for uroplakin was significantly less in affected cats compared with normal cats but not significantly different compared with cats with urolithiasis.[80] It is unclear whether alterations in urothelial markers in cats with idiopathic cystitis represent inherent dysfunction of the urothelium or a secondary response to urothelial injury. Nevertheless, systematic evaluations of protein biomarkers of urothelial differentiation and their role in the pathogenesis of feline idiopathic cystitis as well as their potential as noninvasive diagnostic markers of disease warrant further investigations.

NEUROGENIC INFLAMMATION PARADIGM

Neurogenic inflammation is a process initiated by excitation of small c-fiber sensory afferent neurons and mediated by neuropeptides (eg, substance P, neurokinin, and calcitonin gene-related peptide) released from stimulated nerves.[10,110] Structural or functional defects in the urothelial barrier could permit hydrogen, calcium, and potassium ions, or other urine constituents to come into contact with sensory afferent neurons innervating the urothelium. Alternatively, injury-induced alterations in urothelial release of chemical signaling molecules (eg, ATP, nitric oxide, acetylcholine, substance P, and prostaglandins) may activate sensory afferent neurons and mast cells.[10,73,111] Neurogenic inflammation may also be triggered by histamine and other mediators released by independently activated mast cells in close proximity to neuropeptide-containing sensory neurons.[10,110] Interaction of neuropeptides with tissue receptors results in vasodilation, increased vascular permeability, increased epithelial permeability, increased leukocyte migration, and mast cell activation.[112–115] It is apparent that the combined effects of neuropeptides and mast cell mediators may induce a wide range of biological effects culminating in pain, inflammation, tissue injury, and fibrosis.[10,116] Observations of increased numbers of substance P–containing nerve fibers and their close anatomic association with mast cells in urinary bladders of humans with interstitial cystitis have led to the hypothesis that neurogenic inflammation (and subsequent mast cell activation) represents the common pathway in a multifactorial pathogenesis of human interstitial cystitis.[10,111,117–121]

Similarly, increased numbers of substance P–containing sensory afferent neurons and high affinity substance P receptors have been observed in the bladder submucosa of cats afflicted with chronic idiopathic cystitis.[122] These observations suggest that increased numbers of neuropeptide containing neurons and increased expression of high affinity substance P receptors are associated with inflammation of feline urinary bladders.[82] However, the question of whether these phenomena are a cause or an effect of inflammation and whether they have a role in the etiopathogenesis of feline idiopathic cystitis requires additional investigation.

MAST CELL (NEUROIMMUNE) PARADIGM

When compared with normal cats, increased numbers of mast cells have been identified within the bladder submucosa of some, but not all, cats with idiopathic cystitis.[75,76,80,123] Likewise, mast cell infiltrates are often seen in bladder biopsies obtained from humans with interstitial cystitis.[11,120,124,125] Mast cells secrete a variety of preformed biologically active molecules (histamine, heparin, serotonin, kinins, proteases, phospholipases, chemotactic factors, cytokines, and vasoactive intestinal peptide) as well as molecules synthesized de novo (interleukin-6, leukotrienes, platelet activating factor, prostaglandins, thromboxanes, nitric oxide, tumor necrosis factor-α).[111,120,125] Mast cell secretion can be triggered by anaphylatoxins, antigens, bradykinin, cytokines/lymphokines, hormones, IgE, neurotransmitters, neuropeptides, bacterial toxins, viruses, drugs, and stress.[120,125–127] In addition, release of cytokines from damaged or dysfunctional urothelium is a potent mast cell activator.[120] Products of activated mast cells could be responsible for the inflammation, pain, vasodilation, fibrosis, and smooth muscle contraction associated with human interstitial cystitis and feline idiopathic cystitis.[10,111,120,123,125] Histamine and its metabolites have been found in higher concentrations in the urine of human interstitial cystitis patients and the cystoscopic effluent of cats with idiopathic cystitis.[119,123,128,129]

Despite these observations, the role of mast cells in human interstitial cystitis and feline idiopathic cystitis are unknown. Excessive numbers of mast cells have been observed in bladder biopsies obtained from humans with bladder diseases other than interstitial cystitis, such as, bacterial UTI, neoplasia, outflow obstruction, and stress incontinence.[121,124,125,130] Likewise, the number of mast cells immuno-histochemically stained with c-kit antibody in bladder biopsies obtained from cats with chronic idiopathic cystitis were not significantly different from the number observed in biopsies obtained from cats with urolithiasis.[80] These observations suggest that urinary bladder mastocytosis may not be specific for either human interstitial cystitis or feline idiopathic cystitis. However, electron microscopic studies indicate that the majority of urinary bladder mast cells in humans with interstitial cystitis are activated and are often located in close proximity to neuropeptide-containing sensory nerves. In contrast, mast cell activation is not a feature of lower urinary tract disorders in humans from which interstitial cystitis has been excluded.[117–119,121] The close biochemical and anatomic relationship between urinary bladder mast cells and neuropeptide-containing neurons have led to the hypothesis that neurohormonal triggering of mast cell activation and subsequent release of mast cell mediators play a central role in a multifactorial pathogenesis of human intersitial cystitis.[10,111,118,121] Similar ultrastructural studies of mast cells and their spatial relationship to sensory nerves in cats with idiopathic cystitis have not been performed.

SYSTEMIC PSYCHONEUROENDOCRINE DISEASE PARADIGM

One of the major paradigms shifts over the past decade implicates psychoneuroendocrine dysfunction as a causative factor in the pathogenesis of feline idiopathic cystitis.[20,131,132] Clinical observations suggest that chronic stress induced by environmental, psychologic, physiologic, or comorbid pathologic conditions may play a role in precipitating or exacerbating signs associated with chronic forms of idiopathic cystitis.[133–136] Stress may be defined as any physical, chemical, or emotional force that disturbs or threatens homeostasis, and the accompanying adaptive responses that attempt to restore homeostasis.[137] Although generally beneficial, adaptive responses themselves appear to serve as stressors capable of inducing pathologic changes. Stress has been implicated as a pathologic factor in disease in general, and in autoimmune and neuroinflammatory diseases in particular. It is interesting that stressful events such as earthquakes, seasonal weather changes, moves to a new home, major holidays, and diet changes have been associated with recurrent episodes of lower urinary tract signs in cats.[132,135,136] Other potentially stressful circumstances for cats, such as living in multicat households and inter-cat conflicts, have also been associated with an increased risk of disorders of the lower urinary tract.[133,134,136] Similarly, in humans with interstitial cystitis, stress appears to be a trigger for precipitation or exacerbation of clinical signs.[138]

The association of idiopathic cystitis with environmental, psychologic, physiologic, and pathologic stressors and the identification of multiple abnormalities of the nervous and endocrine systems in affected cats has led to hypothesis that systemic psychoneuroendocrine factors may be involved in the pathogenesis of the disease.[133,139–141] In this paradigm, the urinary bladder is considered to be more likely a victim rather than a perpetrator.[20,131,132] Acute or chronic stress from any source may increase activity of tyrosine hydroxylase (the rate limiting enzyme catalyzing norepinephrine biosynthesis in the pontine locus coeruleus and lead to increased sympathetic autonomic outflow.[142] Observations of increased tyrosine hydroxylase immunoreactivity[140] and plasma norepinephrine concentrations,[84,139] and decreased functional sensitivity of alpha-2-adrenoceptors[143] in cats with chronic idiopathic cystitis are consistent with increased sympathetic drive in affected cats. Activation of the locus coeruleus/noradrenergic system is an important physiologic response to stress; however, it has not been determined whether this response is a cause or consequence of bladder abnormalities observed in cats with chronic idiopathic cystitis.[139,140]

In addition to the locus coeruleus/noradrenergic system, exposure to stress simultaneously activates the hypothalamic-pituitary-adrenal axis (HPAA).[144,145] Stress induced release of glucocorticoids appears to restrain catecholamine synthesis, release, reuptake, and metabolism in the locus coeruleus/noradrenergic system.[145–148] In two small studies of cats with chronic idiopathic cystitis, significant abnormalities of the HPAA were not identified in affected cats, despite having significantly increased plasma norepinephrine concentrations.[84,139] However, in a larger study, significantly decreased plasma cortisol responses to exogenous ACTH and reduction in the size of adrenal glands were observed in cats with chronic idiopathic cystitis compared with healthy cats.[141] Taken together, these observations were interpreted to be indicative of dissociation between the responses of the sympathetic nervous system and hypothalamic-pituitary-adrenal axis to stress in cats with chronic idiopathic cystitis.[84,131,141,144] Furthermore, it was hypothesized that enhanced central noradrenergic drive in the face of inadequate adrenocortical restraint may have a role the disease process.[131,144]

Specific mechanisms by which systemic psychoneuroendocrine disorders in cats may precipitate clinical signs referable to the lower urinary tract apparently have not been identified. Proposed mechanisms include stress-induced central dysregulation of autonomic neurons regulating bladder contraction and stress-induced direct effects on urothelium.[84,144] In cats, the pontine micturition center (aka Barrington's nucleus) refers to an area in the dorsolateral pons and is located adjacent to the locus coeruleus.[149–151] The diversity of afferent and efferent projections to and from Barrington's nucleus indicates that the micturition center functions to integrate pelvic visceral function with behavior. It also provides a balance of inhibitory and excitatory inputs to the sacral parasympathetic neurons that control bladder contractions.[151] The presence of tyrosine hydroxylase–immunoreactive fibers from the locus coeruleus and the high density of glucocorticoid receptors in Barrington's nucleus suggest that stress-induced activation of either the locus coeruleus/adrenergic system or the HPAA may influence micturition.[151–153] Activation of the micturition center via the locus coeruleus/adrenergic system or HPAA could increase excitatory efferent output to pelvic parasympathetic neurons that regulate bladder contraction. Conversely, projections from Barrington's nucleus to the locus coeruleus can also serve as potent activators of the locus coeruleus/noradrenergic system.[151,154] It is conceivable that lower urinary tract disorders that result in chronic stimulation of bladder sensory afferents to Barrington's nucleus may induce persistent activation of the locus coeruleus/noradreneric system.

Alternatively, it has been hypothesized that physiologic responses to stressors may directly affect urothelial integrity.[155] In rodent models, environmental, psychologic, or pharmacologic stressors induced loss of urothelial tight junction integrity, increased paracellular permeability, activation of mast cells, and desquamation of viable superficial urothelial cells.[97,98,127,155,156] In healthy animals, rapid replacement of exfoliated superficial cells and restoration of the urothelial tight junction integrity prevents long-term malfunction of the urothelial barrier.[98] However, long-term increases in the rate of desquamation could have profound effects on urothelial barrier integrity, especially in circumstances where normal urothelial proliferation is inhibited. Although similar studies have not been reported in cats, it is plausible that activation of the sympathetic nervous system and subsequent increases in norepinephrine could increase urothelial permeability by reducing tight junction integrity, thus permitting urine substances greater contact with bladder sensory afferent neurons.[84,157]

Based on psychoneuroendocrine abnormalities identified in affected cats, multi-modal environmental modification (MEMO) strategies designed to minimize reactivity of the stress response system have been advocated as primary therapy for prevention and recurrence of feline idiopathic cystitis.[131,157,158] In an uncontrolled study,[157] 46 client-owned cats living indoors and with a history of recurrent episodes of lower urinary tract signs were managed with individualized plans to reduce environmental and social stressors including changes in physical environment (n=16), increased owner–cat interaction (n=10), moist diet (n=14), enhanced litter box hygiene (n=12), efforts to reduce inter-cat conflict (n=3), and pharmacologic agents (amitriptyline n=7, clomipramine n=1, acepromazine n=2). During the 10-month follow-up period, there was a significant reduction in the frequency of lower urinary tract signs with approximately 70–75% of affected cats remaining symptom free. Unfortunately, the uncontrolled nature of the study and concurrent use of dietary and/or pharmacology interventions in some cats makes it impossible to determine the relative clinical benefits of MEMO. Nevertheless, systematic evaluation of stress factors and their influence on the incidence and pathogenesis of feline idiopathic cystitis and the efficacy of therapeutic strategies designed to mitigate stress in affected cats warrant further investigations.

VIRAL UROPATHOGEN PARADIGM; UPDATE—2008

Despite the fact that viruses have fallen into disfavor as an etiologic paradigm,[20] over the past decade, there has been increasing evidence that FCV may have a causative role in the pathogenesis in at least some cases of feline idiopathic cystitis.[159–161] In the 1980s, transmission electron microscopic examination of urethral matrix- crystalline plugs obtained from male cats with urethral obstruction revealed virus-like particles, similar in size (approximately 25–30 nm) and morphology to caliciviruses (**Fig. 3**).[8,39] These calicivirus-like particles were observed in 38% of 92 urethral plugs obtained from male cats with urethral obstructive idiopathic cystitis.[39] In subsequent studies, an improved virus isolation technique enabled isolation of two new FCV strains (designated FCV-U1 and FCV-U2) from urine obtained from cats with idiopathic cystitis (**Fig. 4**).[161] Genetic analyses revealed that both new urinary FCV strains were genetically distinct from vaccine and other wild-type strains.[161] The observation of calicivirus-like particles in urethral plugs and isolation of two new FCV strains from urine of cats with idiopathic cystitis led the authors to reexamine the role of caliciviruses in feline idiopathic cystitis.

Although isolation of FCV from the urinary tract of affected cats is an essential prerequisite to establishing a "cause and effect" relationship of FCV with idiopathic cystitis, isolation does not necessarily imply causation. Koch's postulates have historically been used to establish a causal relationship between a microorganism and a disease.[162] In recognition of the unique biology of viruses and technological advances in virus identification, however, other investigators have introduced modifications to Koch's postulates.[163] Based on the unified concept of causation proposed by Evans,[163] criteria for establishing a causative relationship between FCV and idiopathic cystitis should include the following: 1) prevalence of the disease should be significantly higher in cats exposed to FCV than in cats not exposed; 2) FCV should be more common in cats with the disease than in cats without the disease when all risk factors are held constant; 3) temporally, the disease should follow exposure to FCV with a distribution of incubation periods on a bell-shaped curve; 4) a spectrum of host responses should follow exposure to FCV along a biological gradient from mild to severe; 5) a measurable host response following exposure to FCV should regularly appear in cats lacking previous exposure or increase in magnitude if previous

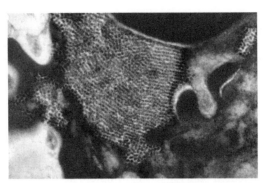

Fig. 3. Transmission electron photomicrograph of a section of matrix-crystalline urethral plug removed from a 3-year-old domestic long-haired cat. Note viruslike particles contained in an unidentified cell (original magnification × 25,600).

exposure occurred; 6) the frequency of induced disease should be higher in cats appropriately exposed to FCV than in those not so exposed; 7) elimination or modification of FCV should decrease the incidence of the disease; and 8) modification of the host's responses on exposure to FCV (eg, effective immunization) should decrease or eliminate the disease.

Large-scale epidemiologic and experimental studies necessary to establish causation have been hindered by lack of a sensitive and rapid means of detecting FCV

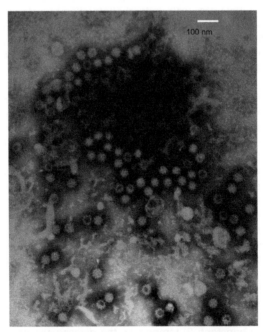

Fig. 4. Transmission electron photomicrograph of feline calcivirus (strain FCV-U2) particles isolated by cell-culture inoculation of urine obtained from a 3-year-old castrated male cat with obstructive idiopathic lower urinary tract disease. Negatively stained with phosphotungstic acid (bar = 100 nm; original magnification × 73,000). (*Photo courtesy of* Dan Taylor, Michigan State University Diagnostic Center for Population and Animal Health.)

urinary tract infections. Because clinical signs, clinical laboratory data, and microscopic evaluation of tissues stained for routine light microscopy cannot reliably distinguish FCV-induced disease from other causes of lower urinary tract signs, the authors developed a FCV p30 gene-based real-time reverse transcription-polymerase chain reaction (RT-PCR) assay optimized for feline urine that is capable of detecting low virus concentrations in urine and a broad range of FCV isolates.[43,44] This RT-PCR assay along with conventional light microscopic methods were used to characterize lower urinary tract disease induced by infection with urinary and respiratory strains of FCV in specific-pathogen free (SPF) cats.[159] FCV was detected by RT-PCR with similar frequency in urinary tract tissues from cats infected with either the urinary or respiratory strain of FCV, and immuno-histochemical staining confirmed localization of FCV antigen to the bladder urothelium. Light microscopy revealed that urinary bladder lesions were more severe and more frequent in cats infected with the urinary strain; oral/respiratory tract lesions were more severe and more frequent in cats infected with the respiratory strain.

In addition, the authors investigated the prevalence of FCV urinary tract infection and FCV antibodies in cats with and without idiopathic cystitis using the FCV RT-PCR assay and a virus neutralizing antibody assay.[160] Study populations included client-owned cats with nonobstructive or obstructive idiopathic cystitis, client-owned or sheltered cats with FCV-induced upper respiratory tract disease, and client-owned or colony-housed healthy asymptomatic cats. FCV nucleic acids were detected with similar frequency (approximately 6%) in urine from cats with nonobstructive or obstructive idiopathic cystitis and cats with upper respiratory tract disease; FCV was not detected in urine from asymptomatic cats. FCV was detected in urine but not in oropharyngeal secretions from three cats with idiopathic cystitis. Mean FCV neutralizing antibody titers for cats with nonobstructive or obstructive idiopathic cystitis and upper respiratory tract disease were significantly higher than the mean titer of asymptomatic control cats. These results confirm urinary shedding of FCV in cats with and without respiratory signs and suggest increased exposure to FCV in cats with idiopathic cystitis compared with asymptomatic controls.

These observations are consistent with the hypothesis that FCV has a causative role in the pathogenesis of at least some cases of feline idiopathic cystitis. Symptomatic disease induced by an infectious agent is the cumulative result of a microorganism's ability to establish infection and compromise host function and, conversely, of a host's ability to resist or curtail infection.[164] Because the virulence of a specific viral uropathogen and the resistance of a given host may vary considerably, FCV urinary tract infections may be asymptomatic or may be associated with substantial morbidity. In general, viral uropathogens may cause disease by: (1) inducing cell injury or death, (2) altering cellular functions, (3) producing toxic compounds or waste products, and (4) stimulating or suppressing an immune response.[164–166] Recent studies have identified the components of the functional receptor for FCV and include the junctional adhesion molecule 1 (JAM-1) and alpha 2,6-linked sialic acid.[167,168] JAM-1 is specifically localized to tight junctions of epithelial and endothelial cells and is involved in regulation of tight junction integrity and permeability, and leukocyte-endothelial cell interactions.[169] Sialic acids are negatively charged sugar molecules usually located at the ends of oligosaccharides attached to glycoproteins, glycolipids, and proteoglycans on the cell surface.[168] It is likely that JAM-1 and sialic acid serve as serotype-independent tissue receptor components capable of mediating virus attachment, infection, and intracellular signaling.[167,168,170] Variations in host receptors may govern host–virus interactions and may play important roles in tissue tropism, organ pathogenesis, and variations observed in host phenotypic expression of infection.

Because urothelial cell tight junctions and GAG layer are integral components of the urothelial barrier, the authors speculate that FCV attachment, infection, and induction of cellular injury or death may alter the structural and/or functional integrity of the urothelium. Subsequent exposure of bladder wall tissues to urine constituents could result in sensory afferent nerve stimulation, mast cell activation, and/or induction of immune-mediated or neurogenic inflammatory responses.[10,73,111] Studies to define the causative role of FCV in the pathogenesis of idiopathic cystitis are in progress.

Summary and Caveats for Future Studies

Since 1996 when the authors assembled the existing body of knowledge about lower urinary tract disease in cats, the understanding of the biological behavior and pathologic features of naturally occurring feline idiopathic cystitis has increased. This increase in knowledge is attributed to results of appropriately designed clinical studies, recognition that laboratory models may provide useful or misleading information, and recognition of the limitations of extrapolating information derived from other species. It is clear that no single model explains all the biological variability observed in cats with idiopathic cystitis. The authors' experience and available evidence indicate that feline idiopathic cystitis represents a syndrome resulting from a number of separate underlying but potentially interrelated mechanisms rather than a disease with a single cause. Identification of safe and effective treatment and prevention strategies of feline idiopathic cystitis will likely vary, depending on the underlying causes.

We are actively seeking identification of causes, combined with results of appropriately controlled studies designed to evaluate the safety and efficacy specific, supportive, and/or symptomatic modes of therapy. Toward this end, future studies designed to identify causative factors and effective treatment strategies should encompass the following principles:

1. Clinical signs of hematuria, dysuria, and pollakiuria may result from fundamentally different causes. There is no single specific diagnostic test or marker that can be relied upon to detect idiopathic cystitis. For patients enrolled in clinical or epidemiologic studies, other causes of lower urinary tract signs must be excluded by use of contemporary diagnostic methods.
2. Various forms of idiopathic cystitis may be encountered in cats with naturally occurring disease (eg, acute self-limiting, chronic persistent or frequently recurrent, or obstructive). Whether these forms represent extremes in the spectrum of clinical manifestations associated with similar etiologic factors, or whether they represent entirely different mechanisms of disease is unknown. Consequently, results of studies preformed in cats with one form of idiopathic cystitis should not necessarily be extrapolated to cats with other forms of the disease.
3. Recurrent clinical signs in patients with idiopathic cystitis are often assumed to be recurrence of the original disease; however, recurrent signs may also be the result of an onset of a different lower urinary tract disease associated with similar clinical signs. This fact should be considered when formulating exclusion and inclusion criteria.
4. Tissues of the lower urinary tract respond to different etiologic agent in a limited number of ways. Meaningful studies must include appropriate control populations to ensure that observed abnormalities are specific for the type of lower urinary tract being studied.
5. Clinical signs subside within 5–7 days without therapy in the majority of cats with idiopathic cystitis. The self-limiting nature of clinical signs in most cats with idiopathic cystitis underscores the need for controlled randomized double-blind

clinical trials rather than anecdotes and opinions when assessing the safely and efficacy of putative therapies.

ILLUSTRATIVE CASE REPORT

A 3 year-old castrated male domestic short hair cat was presented with a 5-day history of acute pollakiuria and dysuria that had progressed to stranguria, vocalizing, and anuria over the past 24 hours. The owner reported no history of any prior illnesses. The cat lived indoors and was fed a 100% dry maintenance diet. Another young female cat had recently been added to the family household. The affected cat was vaccinated for feline calicivirus 24 months ago. Physical examination revealed tachycardia, tachypnea, and a large overdistended painful urinary bladder. Results of a CBC and serum chemical profile were normal. Analysis of a urine specimen collected just before urethral catheterization revealed a urine specific gravity of 1.052, a pH of 7.2 (pH meter), hematuria, proteinuria, and moderate struvite crystalluria. Quantitative culture of urine for aerobic bacteria was negative. Survey abdominal radiographs did not identify any radiopaque uroliths. The cat was anesthetized and urethral patency was restored with a combination of antegrade and retrograde flushing of a crystalline-matrix plug lodged in the distal urethra. Unfortunately, the urethral plug material collected was lost and therefore not available for analysis. Hydration was maintained by intravenous fluid administration and short-term narcotic analgesics were administered. Urethral patency was maintained by placement of a 3.5 French indwelling red rubber urethral catheter. After 24 hours the urinary catheter was removed and empiric antimicrobic therapy was initiated. The cat recovered uneventfully and was discharged 3 days after admission with instructions to feed a struvite calculolytic diet for 30 days. In follow-up studies of samples collected at the time of admission, feline calicivirus nucleic acids were detected by a RT-PCR assay in urine, but not in oropharyngeal secretions.[43,44] A serum FCV neutralizing antibody titer was 1:4096. Once at home, the owner reported that the cat refused to eat the calculolytic diet and therefore was fed its original dry diet. The cat experienced one episode of recurrence of signs of lower urinary tract disease approximately two years later.

Urethral obstruction in cats with idiopathic cystitis may result from: (1) inflammatory swelling of the urethra, (2) urethral muscular spasm, (3) reflex dyssynergia, (4) intraluminal accumulations of sloughed tissue, inflammatory cells, or red blood cells or (5) formation of matrix-crystalline urethral plugs.[18] Physical evidence suggests that formation of a crystalline-matrix urethral plug as sequelae of idiopathic cystitis was responsible, at least in part, for the obstructive uropathy observed in this case. The authors have hypothesized that formation of matrix-crystalline urethral plugs in cats with idiopathic cystitis occur as a result of cystitis-induced increased inflammatory matrix production in conjunction with a concomitant, but etiologically unrelated, crystalluria.[171] Supporting this hypothesis is the observation of recurrent episodes of nonobstructive hematuria and dysuria, and episodes of plug-induced urethral obstruction in other cats with idiopathic cystitis.[18] These observations suggest that male cats with idiopathic cystitis and concomitant crystalluria are at risk for formation of matrix-crystalline urethral plugs and urethral obstruction. The biologic behavior of this case provides evidence that support use of acidifying magnesium-restricted diets to minimize recurrence of matrix-crystalline urethral plugs containing struvite.

Several causative factors may be involved in the pathogenesis of idiopathic cystitis in this case. Introduction of an additional cat into the household could have been a psychological stressor of sufficient magnitude to induce central dysregulation of autonomic neurons regulating bladder contraction and/or directly induced urothelial injury and subsequent signs and sequelae of idiopathic cystitis. Alternatively, detection of FCV in urine and high antibody titer in serum are indicative of an active viral urinary tact infection and suggest that FCV may be causatively involved, either by direct urothelial injury or indirectly as a trigger of neurogenic inflammation or psychoneuroendocrine dysfunction. The authors have detected FCV viruria in a number of cats with idiopathic cystitis without concurrent signs of upper respiratory tract disease or evidence of oral virus shedding.[160,161] Disparities in disease phenotype, tissue tropism, and virus-shedding patterns between FCV strains may be the result of variation in virus virulence, in expression and distribution of host tissue receptors, or in host defense mechanisms. Regardless, detection of FCV viruria and a dramatic concomitant host antibody response support the notion that FCV may be a causative agent in some cases of idiopathic cystitis and emphasize the need for further studies characterizing a cause-and-effect relationship of FCV with idiopathic cystitis.

REFERENCES

1. Buffington CAT, Chew DJ, Kendall MS, et al. Clinical evaluation of cats with non-obstructive urinary tract diseases. J Am Vet Med Assoc 1997;210:46–50.
2. Gerber B, Boretti FS, Kley S, et al. Evaluation of clinical signs and causes of lower urinary tract disease in European cats. J Small Anim Pract 2005;46:571–7.
3. Kruger JM, Osborne CA, Goyal SM, et al. Clinical evaluation of cats with lower urinary tract disease. J Am Vet Med Assoc 1991;199:211–6.
4. Lekcharoensuk C, Osborne CA, Lulich JP. Epidemiologic study of risk factors for lower urinary tract diseases in cats. J Am Vet Med Assoc 2001;218:1429–35.
5. Kalkstein TS, Kruger JM, Osborne CA. Feline idiopathic lower urinary tract disease: part I. Clinical manifestations. Compend Contin Educ Pract Vet 1999;21:15–26.
6. Kruger JM, Osborne CA. Managing feline idiopathic cystitis. In: Bonagura J, Kirk RW, editors. Current veterinary therapy XIV. Philadelphia: WB Saunders Co.; 2009. p. 944–50.
7. Gove PB, editor. Webster's third new international dictionary. Springfield (MA): Merriam-Webster Inc.; 1993. p. 1635.
8. Osborne CA, Kruger JM, Lulich JP, et al. Feline urologic syndrome, feline lower urinary tract disease, feline interstitial cystitis: what's in a name? J Am Vet Med Assoc 1999;214:1470–80.
9. Westropp JL, Buffington CAT. In vivo models of interstitial cystitis. J Urol 2002; 167:694–702.
10. Elbadawi A. Interstitial cystitis: a critique of current concepts with a new proposal for pathologic diagnosis and pathogenesis. Urology 1997;49(Suppl 5A):14–40.
11. Mayer R. Interstitial cystitis pathogenesis and treatment. Curr Opin Infect Dis 2007;20:77–82.
12. Barsanti JA, Finco DR, Scotts EB, et al. Feline urologic syndrome: further investigations into therapy. J Am Anim Hosp Assoc 1982;18:387–90.
13. Kruger JM, Osborne CA. Recurrent, nonobstructive, idiopathic feline lower urinary tract disease: an illustrative case report. J Am Anim Hosp Assoc 1995;31:312–6.
14. Kruger JM, Conway TS, Kaneene JB, et al. Randomized controlled trial of the efficacy of short-term amitriptyline administration for treatment of acute, nonobstructive idiopathic lower urinary tract disease in cats. J Am Vet Med Assoc 2003;222:749–58.
15. Osborne CA, Kruger JM, Lulich JP, et al. Prednisolone therapy of idiopathic feline lower urinary tract disease: a double-blind clinical study. Vet Clin North Am Small Anim Pract 1996;26(3):563–70.

16. Gunn-Moore DA, Shenoy CM. Oral glucosamine and the management of feline idiopathic cystitis. J Feline Med Surg 2004;6:219–25.
17. Markwell PJ, Buffington CAT, Chew DJ, et al. Clinical evaluation of commercially available urinary acidification diets in the management of idiopathic cystitis in cats. J Am Vet Med Assoc 1999;214:361–5.
18. Osborne CA, Kruger JM, Lulich JP, et al. Feline lower urinary tract disease: the Minnesota experience. San Antonio (TX). In: Proceedings of the 15th Annual ACVIM Forum; 1997. p. 338–9.
19. Chew DJ, Buffington CAT, Kendall MS, et al. Amitriptyline treatment for severe recurrent idiopathic cystitis in cats. J Am Vet Med Assoc 1998;213:1282–6.
20. Westropp JL, Buffington CAT, Chew D. Feline lower urinary tract diseases. In: Ettinger SJ, Feldman EC, editors. Textbook of veterinary internal medicine. 6th edition. St. Louis (MO): Elsevier Saunders; 2005. p. 1828–50.
21. Engle GC. A clinical report on 250 cases of feline urological syndrome. Feline Pract 1977;7:24–7.
22. Meier FW. Urethroadenocystitis in the male cat. J Am Vet Med Assoc 1967;151:1059–71.
23. Osbaldiston GW, Taussig RA. Clinical report on 46 cases of feline urological syndrome. Vet Med Small Anim Clin 1970;65:461–8.
24. Mosier JE. Treatment of canine cystitis. J Am Anim Hosp Assoc 1966;2:11–4.
25. Swenson CL, Kruger JM, Gibbons-Burgener SN, et al. Accurate detection of bacteriuria in cats. J Vet Intern Med 2004;18:441.
26. Swenson CL, Boisvert AG, Kruger JM, et al. Evaluation of modified Wright-staining of urine sediment as a method for accurate detection of bacteriuria in dogs. J Am Vet Med Assoc 2004;224:1282–9.
27. Bartges JW, Barsanti JA. Bacterial urinary tract infection in cats. In: Bonagura JD, editor. Kirk's current veterinary therapy XIII small animal practice. Philadelphia: WB Saunders Co.; 2000. p. 880–2.
28. Lees GE. Epidemiology of naturally occurring bacterial urinary tract infections. Vet Clin North Am Small Anim Pract 1984;14:471–9.
29. Barsanti JA, Finco DR, Shotts EB, et al. Feline urologic syndrome: further investigations into etiology. J Am Anim Hosp Assoc 1982;18:391–5.
30. Schechter RD. The significance of bacteria in feline cystitis and urolithiasis. J Am Vet Med Assoc 1970;156:1567–73.
31. Fabricant CG. Herpesvirus-induced urolithiasis in specific-pathogen-free male cats. Am J Vet Res 1977;38:1837–42.
32. Fabricant CG. The feline urological syndrome induced by infection with a cell-associated herpesvirus. Vet Clin North Am 1984;14:493–502.
33. Kruger JM, Osborne CA. The role of viruses in feline lower urinary tract disease. J Vet Intern Med 1990;4:71–8.
34. Fabricant CG, Gillespie JH, Krook L. Intracellular and extracellular mineral crystal formation induced by viral infection of cell cultures. Infect Immun 1971;3:416–9.
35. Fabricant CG, King JM, Gaskin JM, et al. Isolation of a virus from a female cat with urolithiasis. J Am Vet Med Assoc 1971;158:200–1.
36. Gaskell RM, Gaskell CJ, Page W, et al. Studies on a possible etiology for the feline urological syndrome. Vet Rec 1979;105:243–7.
37. Martens JG, McConnell S, Swanson CL. The role of infectious agents in naturally occurring feline urologic syndrome. Vet Clin North Am Small Anim Pract 1984;14:503–11.
38. Shroyer EL, Shalaby MR. Isolation of feline syncytia-forming virus from oropharyngeal swab samples and buffy coat cells. Am J Vet Res 1978;39:555–60.

39. Kruger JM, Osborne CA, Venta PJ, et al. Viral infections of the feline urinary tract. Vet Clin North Am Small Anim Pract 1996;26:281–96.
40. Sutcliffe S, Rohrmann S, Giovannucci E, et al. Viral infections and lower urinary tract symptoms in the third national health and nutrition examination survey. J Urol 2007;178:2181–5.
41. Rich LJ, Fabricant CG. Urethral obstruction in male cats: transmission studies. Can J Comp Med 1969;33:164–5.
42. Rich LJ, Fabricant CG, Gillespie JH. Virus induced urolithiasis in male cats. Cornell Vet 1971;61:542–53.
43. Scansen BA, Kruger JM, Wise AG, et al. In vitro comparison of RNA preparations methods for detection of feline calicivirus in urine in RT-PCR. Am J Vet Res 2005;66:915–20.
44. Scansen BA, Wise AG, Kruger JM, et al. Evaluation of a p30 gene-based real-time reverse transcriptase PCR assay for detection of feline calicivirus. J Vet Intern Med 2004;18:135–8.
45. Gaskin JM, Gillespie JH. Detection of feline syncytia-forming virus carrier state with a micro-immunodiffusion test. Am J Vet Res 1973;34:245–7.
46. German AC, Harbour DA, Helps CR, et al. Is feline foamy virus really a pathogenic? Vet Immunol Immunopathol 2008;123:114–8.
47. Kasza L, Hayward AHS, Betts AO. Isolation of a virus from a cat sarcoma in an established canine melanoma cell line. Res Vet Sci 1969;10:216–8.
48. Pedersen NC, Pool RR, O'Brian T. Feline chronic progressive polyarthritis. Am J Vet Res 1980;41:522–35.
49. Fabricant CG, Gillespie JH. Identification and characterization of a second feline herpesvirus. Infect Immun 1974;9:460–6.
50. Kruger JM, Osborne CA, Goyal, et al. Herpesvirus induced urinary tract infection in SPF cats given methylprednisolone. Am J Vet Res 1990;51:878–85.
51. Kruger JM, Venta PJ, Swenson CL, et al. Prevalence of bovine herpesvirus 4 (BHV-4) infection in cats in central Michigan. J Vet Intern Med 2000;14:593–7.
52. Hansen JS. Urachal remnant in the cat: occurrence and relationship to the feline urologic syndrome. Vet Med Small Anim Clin 1977;67:1090–5.
53. Wilson GP, Dill LS, Goodman RZ. The relationship of urachal defects in the feline urinary bladder to feline urological syndrome. In: Proceedings of the 7th Kal Kan symposium. Vernon (CA): Kal Kan Foods Inc.; 1983. p. 125–9.
54. Noden DM, deLahunta A. The urinary system. In: The embryology of domestic animals. Baltimore (MD): Williams & Wilkins; 1985. p. 312–21.
55. Osborne CA, Johnston GR, Kruger JM, et al. Etiopathogenesis and biological behavior of feline vesicourachal diverticula. Vet Clin North Am Small Anim Prac 1987;17:697–733.
56. Osborne CA, Kroll RA, Lulich JP, et al. Medical management of vesicourachal diverticula in 15 cats with lower urinary tract disease. J Small Anim Pract 1989;30:608–12.
57. Crawford MA. The urinary system. In: Hoskins JD, editor. Veterinary pediatrics: dogs and cats from birth to six months. Philadelphia: WB Saunders Co; 1990. p. 271–92.
58. Fingland RB. Surgery of the urinary bladder. In: Birchard SJ, Sherding RG, editors. Saunder's manual of small animal practice. Philadelphia: WB Saunders Co; 1994. p. 837–8.
59. Osborne CA, Lulich JP, Thumchai R, et al. Feline urolithiasis. Etiology and pathophysiology. Vet Clin North Am 1996;26:217–32.

60. Finco DR, Barsanti JA, Crowell WA. Characterization of magnesium-induced urinary disease in the cat and comparison with feline urologic syndrome. Am J Vet Res 1985;46:391–400.
61. Osborne CA, Abdullahi SU, Polzin DJ, et al. Current status of medical dissolution of canine and feline uroliths. In: Proceedings of the 1983 Kal Kan symposium for the treatment of small animal diseases; 1983. p. 53.
62. Osborne CA, Lulich JP, Kruger JM, et al. Medical dissolution of feline struvite urocystoliths. J Am Vet Med Assoc 1990;196:1053–63.
63. Buffington CA, Rogers QR, Morris JG, et al. Feline struvite urolithiasis: magnesium effect depends on urinary pH. Feline Pract 1985;15:29–33.
64. Jackson JR, Kealy RD, Lawler DF, et al. Long-term safety of urine acidifying diets for cats. Vet Clin Nutr 1995;2:100–7.
65. Lekcharoensuk C, Osborne CA, Lulich JP. Evaluation of trends in frequency of urethrostomy for treatment of urethral obstruction in cats. J Am Vet Med Assoc 2002;221:502–5.
66. Hurst RE, Moldwin RM, Mulholland GS. Bladder defense molecules, urothelial differentiation, urinary biomarkers, and interstitial cystitis. Urology 2007; 69(Suppl 4A):17–23.
67. Parsons CL. The role of the urinary epithelium in the pathogenesis if interstitial cystitis/prostatitis/urethritis. Urology 2007;69(Suppl 4A):9–16.
68. Buffington CAT, Blaisdell JL, Binns SP Jr, et al. Decreased urine glycosaminoglycan excretion in cats with interstitial cystitis. J Urol 1996;155:1801–4.
69. Gao X, Buffington CAT, Au JLS. Effect of interstitial cystitis on drug absorption from urinary bladder. J Pharmacol Exp Ther 1994;271:818–23.
70. Lavelle JP, Meyers SA, Giovani Ruiz W, et al. Urothelial pathophysiological changes in feline interstitial cystitis; a human model. Am J Physiol Renal Physiol 2000;278:F540–53.
71. Apodaca G. The urothelium; not just a passive barrier. Traffic 2004;5:117–28.
72. Lewis SA. Everything you wanted to know about the bladder epithelium but were afraid to ask. Am J Physiol Renal Physiol 2000;278:F867–74.
73. Birder LA. More than just a barrier: urothelium as a drug target for urinary bladder pain. Am J Physiol Renal Physiol 2005;289:F489–95.
74. Lavelle J, Meyers S, Ramage R, et al. Bladder permeability barrier: recovery from selective injury if the surface epithelial cells. Am J Physiol Renal Physiol 2002;283:F242–53.
75. Buffington CA, Chew DJ. Presence of mast cells in submucosa and detrusor of cats with idiopathic lower urinary tract disease. J Vet Intern Med 1993;7:126.
76. Buffington CAT, Chew DJ, Woodworth BE. Animal model of human disease: feline interstitial cystitis. Comp Pathol Bull 1997;29:3–4.
77. Clasper M. A case of interstitial cystitis and Hunner's ulcer in a domestic short hair cat. N Z Vet J 1990;38:158–60.
78. Reche- A Jr, Hagiwara MK. Histopathology and morphometry of urinary bladder of cats with idiopathic lower urinary tract disease. Ciência Rural 2001;31: 1045–9.
79. Specht AJ, Kruger JM, Fitzgerald SD, et al. Light microscopic features of feline idiopathic cystitis. J Vet Intern Med 2003;17:436.
80. Specht AJ, Kruger JM, Fitzgerald SD, et al. Histochemical and immunohistochemical features of chronic feline idiopathic cystitis. J Vet Intern Med 2004; 18:416.
81. Parsons CL, Boychuk D, Jones S, et al. Bladder surface glycosaminoglycans: an epithelial permeability barrier. J Urol 1990;143:139–42.

82. Buffington CAT, Chew DJ, DiBartola SP. Interstitial cystitis in cats. Vet Clin North Am Small Anim Pract 1996;26:317–26.
83. Press SM, Moldwin R, Kushner L, et al. Decreased expression of GP-51 glycosaminoglycan in acts afflicted with feline interstitial cystitis. J Urol 1995;153(Suppl 4):288A.
84. Westropp JL, Kass PH, Buffington CAT. Evaluation of the effects of stress in cats with idiopathic cystitis. Am J Vet Res 2006;67:731–6.
85. Hurst RE, Parsons CL, Roy JB, et al. Urinary glycosaminoglycan as a laboratory marker in the diagnosis of interstitial cystitis. J Urol 1993;149:31–5.
86. Parsons CL, Lilly JD, Stein P. Epithelial dysfunction in non-bacterial cystitis (interstitial cystitis). J Urol 1991;145:732–5.
87. Chelsky MJ, Rosen SI, Knight LC, et al. Bladder permeability in interstitial cystitis is similar to that of normal volunteers: direct measurement by transvesical absorption of 99mtechnetium-diethylenetriaminepentaacetic acid. J Urol 1994; 151:346–9.
88. Dixon JS, Holm-Bentzen M, Gilpin CJ, et al. Electron microscopic investigation of the bladder urothelium and glycocalyx in patients with interstitial cystitis. J Urol 1986;135:621–5.
89. Erickson DR, Ordille S, Martin A, et al. Urinary chondroitin sulfates, heparan sulfate and total sulfated glycosaminoglycans in interstitial cystitis. J Urol 1997;157:61–4.
90. Nickel JC, Emerson C, Cornish J. The bladder mucus (glycosaminoglycan) layer in interstitial cystitis. J Urol 1993;149:716–8, 1993.
91. Nikkila MT. Urinary glycosaminoglycan excretion in normal and stone-forming subjects: significant disturbance in recurrent stone formers. Urol Int 1989;44: 147–59, 1989.
92. Ryall RL, Marshall VR. The value of the 24-hour urine analysis in the assessment of stone-formers attending a general hospital outpatient clinic. Br J Urol 1983;55:1–5.
93. Bade JJ, Laseur M, Nieuwenburg A, et al. A placebo-controlled study of intravesicular pentosanpolysulfate for the treatment of interstitial cystitis. Br J Urol 1997; 79:168–71.
94. Davis EL, El Khoudary SR, Talbott EO, et al. Safety and efficacy of the use of intravesical and oral pentosan polysulfate sodium for interstitial cystitis; a randomized double-blind clinical trial. J Urol 2008;179:177–85.
95. Molholland SG, Hanno P, Parsons CL, et al. Pentosan polysulfate sodium for therapy of interstitial cystitis; a double-blind placebo-controlled clinical study. Urology 1990;35:552–8.
96. Jezernik K, Romih R, Mannherz HG, et al. Immunohistochemical detection of apoptosis, proliferation and inducible nitric oxide synthetase in rat urothelium damaged by cyclophosphamide treatment. Cell Biol Int 2003;27:863–9.
97. Veranič P, Jezernik K. The response of junctional complexes to induced desquamation in mouse bladder urothelium. Biol Cell 2000;92:105–13.
98. Veranič P, Jezernik K. Succession of events in desquamation of superficial urothelial cells as a response to stress induced by prolonged illumination. Tissue Cell 2001;33:280–5.
99. Johansson SL, Fall M. Clinical features and spectrum of light microscopic changes in interstitial cystitis. J Urol 1990;143:1118–24.
100. Rosamilia A, Igawa Y, Higashi S. Pathology of interstitial cystitis. Int J Urol 2003; 10:S11–5.
101. Slobobov G, Feloney M, Gran C, et al. Abnormal expression of molecular markers for bladder impermeability and differentiation in the urothelium of patients with interstitial cystitis. J Urol 2004;171:1554–8.

102. Keay S, Warren JW. A hypothesis for the etiology of interstitial cystitis based on inhibition of bladder epithelial repair. Med Hypotheses 1998;51:79–83.

103. Hauser PJ, Dozmorov MG, Bane BL, et al. Abnormal expression of differentiation related proteins and proteoglycan core proteins in the urothelium of patients with intersitial cystitis. J urol 2008;179:764–9.

104. Laguna P, Smedts F, Nordling J, et al. Keratin expression profiling of transitional epithelium in the painful bladder syndrome/interstitial cystitis. Am J Clin Pathol 2006;125:105–10.

105. Moskowitz MO, Byrne DS, Callahan HJ, et al. Decreased expression of a glycoprotein component of bladder surface mucin (GP1) in interstitial cystitis. J Urol 1994;151:343–5.

106. Keay S, Zhang C-O, Trifillis AL, et al. Decreased 3H-thymidine incorporation by human bladder epithelial cells following exposure to urine from interstitial cystitis patients. J Urol 1996;156:2073–8.

107. Keay S, Seiller-Moiseiwitsch F, Zhang C-O, et al. Changes in human bladder epithelial cell gene expression associated with interstitial cystitis or antiproliferative factor treatment. Physiol Genomics 2003;14:107–15.

108. Keay S, Zhang C-O, Shoenfelt JL, et al. Decreased in vitro proliferation of bladder epithelial cells from patients with interstitial cystitis. Urology 2003;61:1278–84.

109. Zhang C-O, Wang J-Y, Koch KR, et al. Regulation of tight junction proteins and bladder epithelial paracellular permeability by an antiproliferative factor from patients with interstitial cystitis. J Urol 2005;174:2382–7.

110. Jasmin L, Janni G. Experimental neurogenic cystitis. Adv Exp Med Biol 2003;539:319–31.

111. Sant GR, Kempuraj K, Marchand JE, et al. The mast cell in interstitial cystitis: role in pathophysiology and pathogenesis. Urology 2007;69(Suppl 4A):34–40.

112. Church MK, Lowman MA, Rees PH, et al. Mast cells, neuropeptides and inflammation. Agents Actions 1989;27:8–16.

113. Foreman JC. Peptides and neurogenic inflammation. Br Med Bull 1987;43:386–400.

114. McDonald DM. Neurogenic inflammation in the respiratory tracts: actions of sensory nerve mediators on blood vessels and epithelium of the airway mucosa. Am Rev Respir Dis 1987;136:565–72.

115. Payan DG, Levine JD, Goetzl EJ. Modulation of immunity and hypersensitivity by sensory neuropeptides. J Immunol 1984;132:1601–4.

116. Galli SJ. New concepts about the mast cell. N Engl J Med 1993;328:257–65.

117. Elbadawi AE, Light JK. Distinctive ultrastructural pathology of nonulcerative interstitial cystitis: new observations and their potential significance in pathogenesis. Urol Int 1996;56:137–62.

118. LeTourneau R, Pang X, Sant GR, et al. Intragranular activation of bladder mast cells and their association with nerve processes in interstitial cystitis. Br J Urol 1996;77:41–54.

119. Pang X, Boucher W, Triadafilopoulos G, et al. Mast cell and substance P-positive nerve involvement in a patient with both irritable bowel syndrome and interstitial cystitis. Urology 1995;47:436–8.

120. Theoharides TC, Kempuraj D, Sant GR. Mast cell involvement in interstitial cystitis: a review of human and experimental evidence. Urology 2001;57(Suppl 6A):47–55.

121. Theoharides TC, Sant GR, El-Mansoury M, et al. Activation of bladder mast cells in interstitial cystitis: a light and electron microscopic study. J Urol 1995;153:629–36.

122. Buffington CAT, Wolfe- SA Jr. High affinity binding sites for [^{3}H] substance P in urinary bladders of cats with interstitial cystitis. J Urol 1996;160:605–11.

123. Buffington CAT, Chew DJ. Does interstitial cystitis occur in cats?. In: Kirk RW, Bonagura JD, editors. Current veterinary therapy XII. Philadelphia: WB Saunders; 1995. p. 1009–11.

124. Hofmeister MA, Fang H, Ratliff TL, et al. Mast cells and nerve fibers in interstitial cystitis (IC): an algorithm for histologic diagnosis via quantitative image analysis and morphometry (QIAM). Urology 1997;49(Suppl 5A):41–7.

125. Sant GR, Theoharides TC. The role of mast cells in interstitial cystitis. Urol Clin North Am 1994;21:1–53.

126. Lagunoff D, Martin TW, Read G. Agents that release histamine from mast cells. Ann Res Pharmacol Toxicol 1993;23:331–51.

127. Spanos C, Pang X, Ligris K, et al. Stress-induced bladder mast cell activation: implications for interstitial cystitis. J Urol 1997;157:669–72.

128. El-Mansoury M, Boucher W, Sant GR, et al. Increased urine histamine and methylhistamine in interstitial cystitis. J Urol 1994;152:350–3.

129. Holm-Bentzen M, Sondergaard I, Haid T. Urinary excretion of a metabolite of histamine (1,4-methyl-imidazole-acetic acid) in painful bladder disease. Br J Urol 1987;59:230–3.

130. Christmas TJ, Rode J. Characteristics of mast cells in normal bladder, bacterial cystitis and interstitial cystitis. Br J Urol 1991;68:473–8.

131. Buffington CAT. Interstitial cystitis in cats: environmental enrichment and nutrition. In: Proceedings of Hills symposium on lower urinary tract disease. Sunny Isles Beach: 2007. p. 42–4.

132. Buffington CAT, Westropp JL, Chew DJ, et al. Risk factors associate with clinical signs of lower urinary tract disease in indoor-housed cats. J Am Vet Med Assoc 2006;228:722–5.

133. Buffington CAT. External and internal influences on disease risk in cats. J Am Vet Med Assoc 2002;220:994–1002.

134. Cameron ME, Casey RA, Bradshaw JWS, et al. A study of environmental and behavioural factors that may be associated with feline idiopathic cystitis. J Small Anim Pract 2004;45:144–7.

135. Caston HT. Stress and the feline urological syndrome. Feline Pract 1973;4: 14–22.

136. Jones BR, Sanson RL, Morris RS. Elucidating the risk factors of feline urologic syndrome. N Z Vet J 1997;45:100–8.

137. Sternberg EM, Chrousos GP, Wilder RL, et al. The stress response and the regulation of inflammatory disease. Ann Intern Med 1992;117:854–66.

138. Rothrock NE, Lutendorf SK, Kreder KJ, et al. Stress and symptoms in patients with interstitial cystitis. Urology 2001;57:422–7.

139. Buffington CAT, Pacak K. Increased plasma norepinephrine concentration in cats with interstitial cystitis. J Urol 2001;165:2051–4.

140. Reche- A Jr, Buffington CAT. Increased tyrosine hydroxylase immunoreactivity in the locus coeruleus of cats with interstitial cystitis. J Urol 1998;159: 1045–8.

141. Westropp JL, Welk KA, Buffington CAT. Small adrenal glands in cats with feline interstitial cystitis. J Urol 2003;170:2494–7.

142. Bremner JD, Krystal JH, Southwick SM, et al. Noradrenergic mechanisms in stress and anxiety: I. Preclinical studies. Synapse 1996;23:28–38.

143. Westropp JL, Kass PH, Buffington CAT. In vivo evaluation of α_2-adrenoceptors in cats with idiopathic cystitis. Am J Vet Res 2007;68:203–7.

144. Buffington CA. Comorbidity if interstitial cystitis with other unexplained clinical conditions. J Urol 2004;172:1242–8.
145. Kvetnansky R, Pacak K, Fukuhara K, et al. Sympathoadrenal system in stress: interaction with hypothalamic-pituitary-adrenocortical system. Ann N Y Acad Sci 1995;771:131–58.
146. Fukuhara K, Kvetnansky R, Cizza G, et al. Interrelations between sympathoadrenal system and hypothalamo-pituitary-adrencortical/thyroid systems in rats exposed to cold stress. J Neuroendocrinol 1996;8:533–41.
147. Kvetnansky R, Fukuhara K, Pacak K, et al. Endogenous glucocorticoids restrain catecholamine synthesis and release at rest and during immobilization stress in rats. Endocrinology 1993;133:1411–9.
148. Makino S, Smith MA, Gold PW. Regulatory role of glucocorticoids and glucocorticoid receptor mRNA levels on tyrosine gene expression in the locus coeruleus during repeated immobilization stress. Brain Res 2002;943:216–23.
149. Barrington FJF. The effect of lesions of the hind- and mid-brain on micturition in the cat. Q J Exp Physiol 1925;15:81–102.
150. Blok BF, Holstege G. The central nervous system control of micturition in cats and humans. Behav Brain Res 1998;92:119–25.
151. Valentino RJ, Miselis RR, Pavcovich LA. Pontine regulation of pelvic viscera: pharmacologic target for pelvic visceral dysfunctions. Trends Pharmacol Sci 1999;20:253–60.
152. Valentino RJ, Page ME, Luppi P–H, et al. Evidence for widespred afferents to Barrington's nucleus, a brainstem region rich in corticotropin-releasing hormone neurons. Neuroscience 1994;62:125–43.
153. Lechner SM, Valentino RJ. Glucocorticoid receptor-immunoreactivity in corticotropin-releasing factor afferents to the locus coeruleus. Brain Res 1999;816:17–28.
154. Valentino RJ, Chen S, Zhu Y, et al. Evidence for divergent projections to the brain noradrenergic system and the spinal parasympathetic system from Barrington's nucleus. Brain Res 1996;732:1–15.
155. Ercan F, San T, Cavdar S. The effects of cold-restraint stress on urinary bladder wall compared with interstitial cystitis morphology. Urol Res 1999;27:454–61.
156. Dalal E, Medalia O, Harari O, et al. Moderate stress protects female mice against bacterial infection of the bladder by eliciting uroepithelial shedding. Infect Immun 1994;62:5505–10.
157. Buffington CAT, Westropp JL, Chew DJ, et al. Clinical evaluation of multimodal environmental modification (MEMO) in the management of cats with idiopathic cystitis. J Feline Med Surg 2006;8:261–8.
158. Westropp JL, Buffington CAT. Feline idiopathic cystitis: current understanding of pathophysiology and management. Vet Clin North Am Small Anim Pract 2004;34:1043–55.
159. Kruger JM, Pfent CP, Clark AK, et al. Feline calicivirus-induce urinary tract disease in specific-pathogen-free cats. J Vet Intern Med 2007;21:684.
160. Larson J, Kruger JM, Wise AG, et al. Epidemiology of feline calicivirus urinary tract infection in cats with idiopathic cystitis. J Vet Intern Med 2007;21:684.
161. Rice CC, Kruger JM, Venta PJ, et al. Genetic characterization of 2 novel feline caliciviruses isolated from cats with idiopathic lower urinary tract disease. J Vet Intern Med 2002;16:293–302.
162. Koch R. Ueber bakteriologische Forschung. In: "Verh. X Int. Med. Congr, Berlin, 1890." Berlin: August Hirschwald; 1892. p. 35.
163. Evans AS. Causation and disease: the Henle-Koch postulates revisited. Yale J Biol Med 1976;49:175–95.

164. Lichtenburg F. Infectious disease. In: Cotran RS, Kumar V, Robbins SL, editors. Pathologic basis of disease. 4th edition. Philadelphia: WB Saunders; 1989. p. 307–15.
165. Sosnovtsev SV, Prikhod'ko EA, Belliot G, et al. Feline calicivirus replication induces apoptosis in cultured cells. Virus Res 2003;94:1–10.
166. Willcocks MM, Carter MJ, Roberts LO. Cleavage of eukaryotic initiation factor eIF4G and inhibition of host-cell protein synthesis during feline calicivirus infection. J Gen Virol 2004;85:1125–30.
167. Makino A, Shimojima M, Miyazawa T, et al. Junctional adhesion molecule 1 is a functional receptor for feline calicivirus. J Virol 2006;80:4482–90.
168. Stuart AD, Brown TDK. α2,6-Linked sialic acid acts as a receptor for feline calicivirus. J Gen Virol 2007;88:177–86.
169. Ebnet K, Suzuki A, Ohno S, et al. Junctional adhesion molecules (JAMs): more molecules with dual functions? J Cell Sci 2004;117:19–29.
170. Barton ES, Forrest JC, Connolly JL, et al. Junction adhesion molecule is a receptor for reovirus. Cell 2001;104:441–51.
171. Osborne CA, Kruger JM, Lulich JP, et al. Feline matrix-crystalline plugs: a unifying hypothesis of causes. J Small Anim Pract 1992;33:172–7.

Changing Paradigms in the Frequency and Management of Canine Compound Uroliths

Lisa K. Ulrich, CVT*, Carl A. Osborne, DVM, PhD,
Amy Cokley, BS, Jody P. Lulich, DVM, PhD

KEYWORDS

• Urolith • Compound • Mixed • Struvite • Calcium oxalate

WHAT ARE COMPOUND UROLITHS?

Most uroliths are composed of a predominant mineral type (>70%) mixed with lesser quantities of other minerals. One or more mineral types may also be admixed within layers of a urolith. If mineral types do not comprise greater than 70% of a layer, it is classified as a mixed urolith (**Fig. 1**). If different minerals are separated into distinct juxtaposed bands or layers, and if one portion of the urolith comprises at least 70% of one mineral type and is surrounded by one or more layers composed primarily (>70%) of a different mineral, it is classified as a compound urolith (**Fig. 2**). For example, a urolith composed of 100% calcium oxalate on the interior, surrounded by predominantly struvite on the exterior, would be classified as compound (**Fig. 3**). Similarly, a dog with a silica urocystolith that subsequently develops a urease-producing bacterial urinary tract infection may form a shell of struvite surrounding the silica. This urolith would also be classified as compound (**Fig. 4**).

Uroliths may also be classified as compound if the nidus, stone, shell, surface crystals, bands, or focal deposits fit the criteria described above (see **Fig. 2**). The compound classification may also be used for uroliths composed predominantly (>70%) of different mineral types retrieved from different locations in the urinary tract. For example, a dog with calcium oxalate renoliths that subsequently develops a urinary

---

This article has been supported in part by an educational gift from Hill's Pet Nutrition, Topeka, Kansas.

Veterinary Clinical Sciences Department, Minnesota Urolith Center, College of Veterinary Medicine, University of Minnesota, 1352 Boyd Avenue, St. Paul, MN 55108, USA

* Corresponding author.

E-mail address: unger003@umn.edu (L.K. Ulrich).

doi:10.1016/j.cvsm.2008.09.009
0195-5616/08/$ – see front matter © 2008 Elsevier Inc. All rights reserved.
vetsmall.theclinics.com

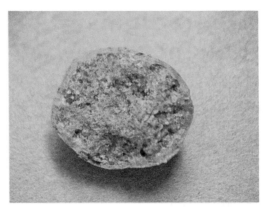

Fig. 1. Urolith classified as mixed. Sample is composed of 55% ammonium urate and 45% struvite, from an 11-month-old female, spayed Yorkshire terrier.

tract infection with a urease-positive bacteria may form predominantly struvite urocystoliths.

Diametrically opposed mineral types may also be found within the same location of the urinary tract (**Fig. 5**). Studies of human beings with bilateral nephroliths also document that significant differences in urolith composition can be present at the same time.[1]

HOW FREQUENTLY ARE COMPOUND UROLITHS OBSERVED?

Compound uroliths comprised 9.1% of canine uroliths submitted to the Minnesota Urolith Center (MUC) in 2007. During the same period, compound uroliths comprised 3.2% of feline uroliths. We have reported the prevalence of canine compound uroliths previously as 6.5%, from 1981 to 1996, and 8% in 2002.[2,3] Reports from other veterinary stone centers have excluded compound and mixed uroliths from their totals.[4,5] The exclusion of these urolith types diminishes the importance of recognizing the unique causal factors that may be present in each individual patient.

WHY IS IT IMPORTANT TO RECOGNIZE COMPOUND UROLITHS?

The compiled prevalence of canine compound uroliths in our series from 1981 to 2007 was 8.8%. Although this is not a large percentage of our total urolith submissions, it is

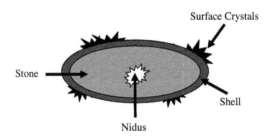

Fig. 2. Cross-section of a urolith, with representation of separate areas that may be present. Nidus: the area of obvious initiation of urolith growth, which is not necessarily the geometric center of the sample. Stone: the major body of the urolith. Shell: a complete outer concentric lamination of the urolith. Surface crystals: an incomplete outer lamination of the urolith.

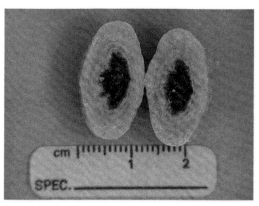

Fig. 3. Calcium oxalate inner layer, struvite outer layer. Patient is a female, spayed 9-year-old Dachshund.

of importance when formulating management strategies to dissolve stones or minimize their recurrence. Likewise, knowledge of mineral types is helpful in predicting efficacy of lithotripsy, as the composition of the urolith may affect the fragility and thus the effectiveness of this procedure.[6]

HOW DO COMPOUND UROLITHS FORM?

Compound uroliths are likely to form when factors initially promoting precipitation of one type of mineral are superceded by factors promoting precipitation of a different mineral. For example, antibiotics and urine acidifiers are often used to manage infection-induced struvite uroliths. The antibiotics may eradicate or suppress microbial urease, reducing precipitation of struvite. However, acidosis associated with urinary acidifiers or acidifying diets may promote hypercalciuria, resulting in a shell of calcium oxalate or calcium phosphate that surrounds the nidus of struvite (**Fig. 6**).

Uroliths that have formed around foreign material in the urinary tract can also be classified as compound. The authors have observed suture material, urinary catheters, metal pellets, plant material, hair strands, and other foreign objects within uroliths

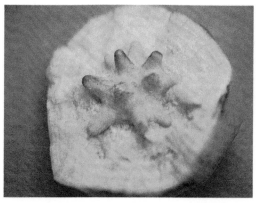

Fig. 4. Silica inner layer, struvite outer layer. Patient is a mixed breed 8-year-old male, castrated dog.

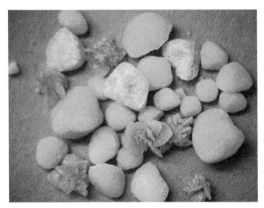

Fig. 5. Rosette-shaped uroliths are composed of calcium oxalate; smooth surfaced uroliths are composed of struvite. Uroliths all removed surgically from the bladder of a 10-year-old male, castrated Yorkshire terrier.

of various mineral types (**Figs. 7** and **8**). The presence of foreign material within the urinary tract of canine stones has also been reported by other investigators.[7,8]

Drugs used to manage urinary tract infections can also form crystals in the urine and become incorporated into the urolith. In 2007, in the authors' compound urolith series, five cases of calcium oxalate, struvite, or purine uroliths surrounded by crystals of sulfa metabolites were found (**Fig. 9**). Also in 2007, eight patients with uroliths surrounded by outer layers composed of fluoroquinolone crystals were detected (**Fig. 10**).

WHAT PROTOCOLS CAN BE USED TO ELIMINATE COMPOUND UROLITHS?

Risk factors that predispose the patient to precipitation of different minerals in compound uroliths are usually complex. Therefore, designing effective medical protocols to manage them can be a unique challenge. Dissolution protocols have been developed to manage struvite, ammonium urate, and cystine uroliths.[9] One strategy to manage compound uroliths suspected to have an outer layer of mineral conducive

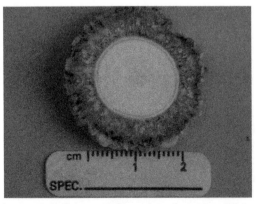

Fig. 6. Majority of the interior of the urolith consists of struvite. Calcium oxalate predominates in the outer layer. Urolith from a 12 year-old female spayed miniature Schnauzer.

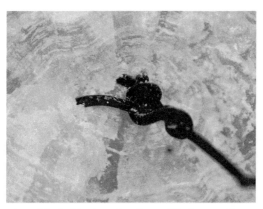

Fig. 7. Suture as a foreign object nidus in a struvite urolith from an 8-year-old female, spayed Yorkshire terrier.

to dissolution is to design a protocol to dissolve the outer layer first. Serial re-evaluation of the size of the compound urolith by an appropriate imaging technique is recommended. Once there is no further reduction in urolith size, medical therapy may be adjusted to attempt dissolution of suspected minerals in the inner layers.

Alternatively, the authors have reduced the size of compound uroliths by dissolving outer layers, followed by removing the remaining smaller portion by voiding urohydro-propulsion. Symptomatic compound uroliths that are refractory to medical protocols should be removed by lithotripsy or surgery. In some patients with asymptomatic uroliths, a "wait and see" strategy, with periodic assessment of changes in urolith size determined by imaging techniques, may be an option.

HOW CAN RECURRENCE OF COMPOUND UROLITHS BE MINIMIZED?
General Recommendations

In most cases, prevention protocols are designed to minimize recurrence of minerals that comprise the center, rather than the outer layers, of compound uroliths. This recommendation is based on the concept of heterogeneous nucleation. In this concept, a greater urine concentration of lithogenic minerals is required for uroliths to spontaneously precipitate in the absence of solid surfaces within the lumen of the

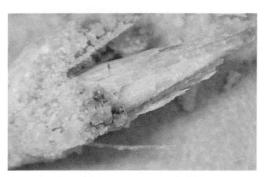

Fig. 8. Plant material as a foreign object core surrounded by struvite in a urolith surgically removed from a 3-year-old male, castrated miniature Poodle.

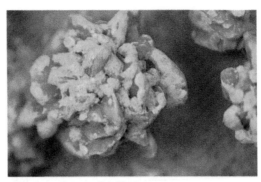

Fig. 9. Urolith composed of calcium oxalate with outer surface crystals of a sulfa metabolite.

urinary tract (homogenous nucleation), than is required for uroliths to precipitate around a pre-existing solid structure (eg, suture material, catheters, and pre-existing uroliths of a different mineral type). In the context of compound uroliths, logic suggests that the initial core composed of one mineral type and formed by homogeneous nucleation contributed to the formation of outer layers of a different mineral type formed by heterogeneous nucleation. Therefore, minimizing risk factors for precipitation of minerals found in the core would eliminate heterogeneous nucleation and, thus, would minimize precipitation of minerals found in the outer layers of the urolith (ie, it would increase the formation product).

Supersaturation of urine with minerals is a prerequisite for urolith formation. It follows that increased water intake would logically lead to reduction in urine concentration of lithogenic minerals, thus minimizing recurrence of all types of uroliths. In addition to reducing the concentration of lithogenic minerals, formation of large volumes of less-concentrated urine decreases the risk of urolithiasis by increasing the frequency of micturition and, thus, the frequency that crystals are voided. To minimize formation of concentrated urine, the authors recommend feeding high-moisture canned foods. Alternatively, water can be added to dry diets with the goal of achieving a urine-specific gravity value of less than 1.020. In general, the authors avoid indiscriminate use of diuretics because of their propensity for adverse effects (eg,

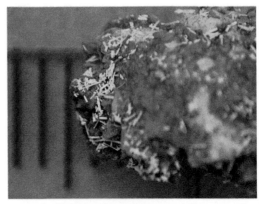

Fig. 10. Urolith composed of calcium oxalate with outer surface crystals of a fluoroquinolone drug. Sample removed from an 8-year-old Maltese dog.

dehydration, hypokalemia, hypercalcemia, and increased urinary excretion of some lithogenic minerals). Addition of supplemental sodium chloride to stimulate thirst should be avoided for similar reasons.

Specific Recommendations

Compound uroliths containing a core of calcium oxalate monohydrate or calcium oxalate dihydrate, or both, were the most common interior mineral type in canine uroliths in 2007 in the authors' series. This type of compound urolith comprised 1369 out of 3236 compound uroliths submitted (42.3%) (**Table 1**).

CALCIUM OXALATE NIDUS
Struvite Outer Layer

The most common compound uroliths in the authors' series are those with an inner layer of calcium oxalate surrounded by an outer layer composed of struvite: 1183 of the 3236 (35%) compound canine uroliths in 2007 (see **Fig. 3**).

The paradox in managing patients forming compound uroliths composed of different layers of calcium oxalate and struvite is that attempts to minimize risk factors for struvite urolith formation (such as reducing urine pH, and the urine concentration of magnesium and phosphorus) may increase the risk for calcium oxalate urolith formation. In this situation, the authors recommend that emphasis be placed on minimizing recurrence of calcium oxalate uroliths, because calcium oxalate uroliths cannot be dissolved medically. In contrast, struvite uroliths that form secondary to infections with urease-producing microbes can often be dissolved by medical protocols. For uroliths containing a core of calcium oxalate surrounded by a shell of infection-induced struvite, it is logical to assume that an initial episode of calcium oxalate uroliths predisposed the patient to infection-induced struvite uroliths. Therefore, preventative management should include efforts to eradicate or control recurrent urinary tract infections in conjunction with medical management designed to minimize calcium oxalate formation.

Calcium Phosphate Outer Layer

In 59 out of 3236, or 1.8% of compound uroliths in the authors' series, a shell of calcium phosphate surrounded a core of calcium oxalate. The authors hypothesize that excessive calcium excretion was a primary abnormality in these dogs. Therefore, the authors formulate prevention strategies based on the principles designed for uroliths composed entirely of calcium oxalate.

Purine Outer Layer

Some compound uroliths (24 out of 3236, or 0.7% in the authors' series) contained a core of calcium oxalate and a shell of urate salts. Consumption of diets moderately reduced in protein and that promote formation of alkaline urine (eg, the type of diet commonly recommended to manage calcium oxalate) are also recommended for prevention of purine uroliths.

Compound uroliths containing a core of magnesium ammonium phosphate hexahydrate (struvite), were the second most common interior mineral type in canine uroliths in the 2007 series. Of the 3236 of the compound canine uroliths analyzed at the MUC laboratory in 2007, 1311 or 40.5% contained a core of struvite (see **Table 1**).

Mineral salts surrounding struvite include calcium oxalate (229 of 3236, or 7%), purines (113 of 3236, or 3.5%), calcium hydrogen phosphate dihydrate, commonly called "brushite" (38 of 3236, or 1.2%), and silica (12 of 3236, or 0.4%). For all of these mineral types surrounding struvite, the likelihood of a urinary tract infection initiating

48 Ulrich et al

Table 1
Distribution of 3236 canine compound uroliths received at the Minnesota Urolith Center in 2007

Core Minerals[a]	Calcium Oxalate	Magnesium Ammonium Phosphate (Struvite)	Purines[b]	Calcium Phosphate	Calcium Hydrogen Phosphate Trihydrate (Brushite)	Magnesium Phosphate Hydrate	Uric acid Monohydrate[c]	Silica	Cystine	Xanthine	Fluoro-Quinolone Drug	Magnesium Hydrogen Phosphate (Newberyite)[d]	Sulfa Drug	Total
Calcium oxalate	NA	1183	24	59	52	3	4	36	3	2	2	0	1	1369
Magnesium ammonium phosphate (struvite)	229	NA	113	905	38	0	0	12	1	1	5	4	3	1311
Purines[b]	72	132	NA	3	0	0	0	6	2	0	1	0	1	217
Calcium phosphate	67	92	1	NA	15	0	0	0	1	0	0	2	0	178
Brushite	11	0	0	3	NA	0	0	0	0	0	0	0	0	14
Uric acid monohydrate[c]	15	4	0	0	0	0	NA	0	0	0	0	0	0	19
Silica	92	16	1	—	0	1	0	NA	2	0	0	0	0	112
Cystine	4	1	0	0	0	0	0	1	NA	0	0	0	0	6
Xanthine	1	0	0	0	0	0	0	0	0	NA	0	0	0	1
Foreign body	1	8	0	0	0	0	0	0	0	0	0	0	0	9
Total	492	1436	139	970	105	4	4	55	9	3	8	6	5	3236

Actual number of canine uroliths classified as compound in 2007 was 3698. Approximately 450 uroliths were composed of mineral combinations too complex for simple classification: for example, a urolith with the composition central nidus of calcium oxalate, surrounded by a stone of struvite, encased on an outer shell of calcium oxalate.
[a] Quantitative analysis by polarizing light microscopy or infra-red spectroscopy.
[b] Including ammonium urate, uric acid, sodium urate, salts of uric acid.
[c] Uric acid monohydrate is suspected to be a mineral formed by pets consuming diets contaminated with melamine and cyanuric acid.
[d] Likely induced by preservation in formalin.

urolith formation necessitates monitoring for, and preventing future urinary tract infections. A twofold management strategy should also include selecting a canned or moist diet designed to minimize the risk factors associated with each particular outer mineral type.

STRUVITE NIDUS
Calcium Phosphate Outer Layer

Calcium phosphate (primarily the carbonate-apatite form) was the most common mineral found in the outer layers surrounding cores of struvite. In the authors' series, 905 of the 3236 compound uroliths (28%) were struvite stones surrounded by calcium phosphate outer layers. This type of compound urolith has more than doubled in prevalence since last reported in 1998, at which time it comprised 13%. This combination is predictable because struvite and calcium phosphate uroliths share several common risk factors. For example, the solubility of both salts is reduced in alkaline urine. In addition, increasing urine phosphate concentration increases the risk of formation of both types of minerals. Precipitation of struvite and calcium phosphate are promoted by urinary tract infections, with urease-producing microbes that hydrolyze urea into ammonia and carbonate; ammonia is a component of struvite uroliths and carbonate is a component of calcium phosphate (carbonate-apatite) uroliths.

Fortunately, most recommendations to minimize struvite urolith recurrence also minimize formation of calcium phosphate. Treatment with appropriate antimicrobics to eradicate or control urinary tract infections caused by urease-producing microbes is essential. Reducing dietary protein with the goal of reducing the urine concentration of urea will minimize the quantity of ammonia generated by microbial urease. In addition, reduction of dietary protein also minimizes renal medullary urea and thus promotes polyuria.

When using diets designed to acidify the urine, what factors should be considered? On the one hand, because reduction of urine calcium excretion is emphasized in the management of calcium oxalate uroliths, acidification of urine would minimize the quantity of ionic phosphate available to form struvite and ammonium phosphate. On the other hand, however, chronic acidification would promote urine calcium excretion and thus increase the risk for formation of uroliths containing calcium.[9] When fed to dogs as a part of a struvite-dissolution protocol, diets designed to promote acid urine may be a risk factor for calcium-containing mineral types. Attempts to acidify urine of dogs with pre-existing struvite uroliths may be one factor that helps to explain why calcium-containing minerals surrounded 340 of 1311 compound uroliths containing a core of struvite (229 calcium oxalate, 59 calcium phosphate, 52 brushite) (see **Fig. 6**).

Calcium Oxalate Outer Layer

The most common mineral associated with silica was calcium oxalate (92 of the 112, or 82% of silica compound stones were surrounded by calcium oxalate). Perhaps one common denominator linking these two minerals is consumption of plant-based foods that contain more silisic and oxalic acid than animal-based foods. In addition, one mineral may serve as a template for precipitation for the other (a phenomenon called "epitaxy").

Protocols to minimize silica urolith recurrence have been devised on the basis of logic. Diets containing substantial quantities of corn gluten feed, soybean hulls, and rice hulls typically contain large quantities of silisic acid and have been associated with silica uroliths. Diets containing these ingredients also have increased quantities of oxalic acid. Therefore, the authors recommend that diets containing substantial quantities of plant proteins be avoided. When calcium oxalate or urate surrounds a core of silica, strategies for prevention of the outer calcium oxalate layer are usually compatible with a reduction in risk factors for silica urolith formation. When compound uroliths with a core of silica have an outer layer of struvite, recurrent urinary tract infections should also be eliminated or controlled.

CALCIUM PHOSPHATE CORE: VARIABLE OUTER LAYER

A a core of calcium phosphate was observed in 178 out of 3236 (5%) of compound uroliths in the authors' series. They were the most often surrounded either by shells of calcium oxalate (67 of 178) or struvite (92 of 178). These uroliths can be managed in a fashion similar to uroliths with cores of calcium oxalate or struvite and outer layers of calcium phosphate.

PURINE CORE: VARIABLE OUTER LAYER

When purines, such as ammonium urate, sodium urate, uric acid, or other salts of uric acid, are found in either the interior or exterior layers of a urolith, the authors' first recommendation is to investigate the possibility of liver disease or dysfunction, such as a portal vascular anomaly. Only 217 of 3236 compound uroliths (6.7%) in the authors' series contained a core of purines. Of those surrounded by a shell of struvite (132 of 3236), it is probable that the purine core predisposed the patient to a urinary tract infection with urease-producing microbes, which in turn promoted formation of struvite. Strategies to prevent recurrence of this type of compound urolith should include eradication or control of urinary tract infections in addition to protocols designed to prevent recurrence of purine uroliths. This includes feeding diets moderately reduced in protein that promote formation of alkaline urine.

The authors' recommendations for management of purine uroliths surrounded by a shell of calcium oxalate also consist of feeding diets moderately reduced in protein that promote formation of alkaline urine. These types of diets are commonly recommended to manage calcium oxalate uroliths, as well as prevention of purine uroliths.

XANTHINE CORE: VARIABLE OUTER LAYER

Two dogs formed compound uroliths containing xanthine in the outer shell layer (both were being treated with allopurinol). Also observed was a compound urolith containing a core of xanthine in a urolith retrieved from a dog. It was not determined whether this dog was being administered allopurinol. Unfortunately, as the urine concentration of uric acid declines in response to allopurinol therapy, the concentrations of hypoxanthine and xanthine increases. The magnitude of xanthinuria increases in proportion to the quantity of purines in the diet and the dose and frequency of allopurinol administration. Prevention of recurrence encompasses reduction of dietary purines and discontinuing or reducing the dose of allopurinol.

FOREIGN OBJECT CORE

Foreign objects were found as a core in 105 out of 40,612 (0.25%) canine uroliths in the year 2007. Suture material was the most common foreign object, detected in 74 out of 105 foreign object cores (see **Fig. 7**). Suture material was most commonly surrounded by struvite (35 of 105, and calcium oxalate in 25 of 105). In cases having a suture or suspected suture nidus, the authors hypothesize that these patients have had a history of urolithiasis. A documented previous urolith episode was verified in 73 of 105 (70%) patients with a suture nidus. Urolithiasis tends to be recurrent, particularly if preventative measures are not initiated. Patients with uroliths containing a suture foreign object core have historically formed uroliths, and may be at risk for future urolith formation. In these suture nidus cases, the authors have observe metabolic and infection-induced mineral types surrounding the suture core.

PLANT FOREIGN OBJECT

Plant material (plant awns or other plant material) was identified in 5 out of 40,612 canine stones in 2007 (see **Fig. 8**). In all cases, the plant material was surrounded by an outer layer of struvite. None of the five dogs was reported to have had a previous episode of urolithiasis. Just how plant awns or other plant material gain access to the lumen of the urinary bladder is often subject of conjecture.[7] These patients may not have a previous history of urolithiasis. The struvite surrounding the plant material likely is a result of urinary tract infection promoted by the foreign object nidus.

HOLLOW CYLINDRICAL CENTRAL AREA

In addition to obvious suture material, the authors often have observed uroliths containing hollow cylindrical central areas. The authors hypothesize that these unique structures are the result of dissolved suture material (**Fig. 11**). In 2007, the authors observed 352 canine uroliths containing a hollow cylindrical central area or areas. Calcium oxalate was by far the most common outer mineral type, detected in 272, or 72% of the 352 samples with a hollow cylindrical area. In 33 (9.3%) of the 352 uroliths containing a hollow central area, a thin band lining the hollow area was found, with an outer layer of struvite (**Fig. 12**). Of the 353 dogs with uroliths containing a hollow cylindrical central area, 315, or 89% were reported to have had a previous urolith episode. This observation supports the hypothesis that this hollow cylindrical central area was originally occupied by sutures. Selection and use of appropriate suture material for the urinary tract would minimize exposure of suture material to the lumen of the urinary tract, thus eliminating a potential nidus for crystal formation.

HOW SHOULD RESPONSE TO THERAPY BE MONITORED?

Treatment of compound uroliths often necessitates combining several unrelated treatment regimens; therfore, diligent monitoring of the efficacy and safety of the selected

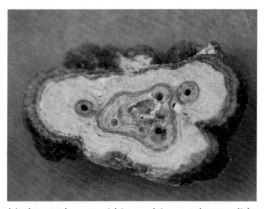

Fig. 11. Hollow cylindrical central areas within a calcium oxalate urolith removed from a 10-year-old male, castrated Jack Russell terrier.

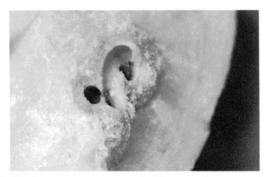

Fig. 12. Hollow cylindrical central area surrounded by a band composed of calcium oxalate. The outer layers of the urolith are composed of struvite. Urolith removed from a 9-year-old female, spayed Pomeranian.

therapy is especially important. Control of urolith-forming risk factors should result in reduction of urine concentration (eg, specific gravity) and reduction or elimination of crystalluria. The authors recommend urinalyses be repeated at appropriate intervals to determine if treatment protocols are associated with desired outcomes. Consideration of collection technique, storage time, and preservation method are important in interpreting in vivo versus in vitro crystalluria. Delays in analysis may cause in vitro preciptation of crystals that do not reflect in vivo conditions.[10]

WHAT IF UROLITHS RECUR DESPITE PREVENTION ATTEMPTS?

Because diet modification and drug therapy usually do not eliminate all underlying risk factors, it is unrealistic to expect complete prevention of recurrent urolithiasis. In the authors' experience, appropriate therapy eliminates urolith recurrence in some dogs and minimizes urolith recurrence in others. Postsurgical imaging procedures to ensure complete removal of uroliths is a standard of patient care. Unfortunately, this aspect of surgical treatment is sometimes ignored. Detection of uroliths weeks or months later results in the phenomenon that the authors call "pseudo-recurrence."[11]

Recurrence of uroliths does not always mean that additional surgical therapy is required. To reduce the need for additional surgery, schedule follow-up evaluations to facilitate detection of urocystoliths when they are small enough to pass easily through the urethral lumen. Small urocystoliths can often be easily removed by voiding urohydropropulsion or other minimally invasive techniques. If patients are re-evaluated only when they develop clinical signs typical of urolith recurrence, the uroliths often have become too large to pass through the urethra. Appropriately scheduled re-examinations also promote client compliance with preventative therapy.

SUMMARY

The compiled prevalence of canine compound uroliths in the authors' series from 1981 to 2007 was 8.8%. Although this does not comprise a large percentage of the total canine urolith submissions to the MUC laboratory, it is of importance when formulating management strategies for individual patients to either dissolve existing stones or minimize urolith recurrence.

Further investigation to identify the contributory factors in compound urolith formation may highlight causal factors. For example, the rise in incidence of calcium-containing outer layers surrounding struvite uroliths may be attributable to the use of acidifying diets administered with the goal of managing struvite urolithiasis. The authors plan to continue to monitor epidemiologic trends of compound uroliths as they focus their mission to make the surgical removal of uroliths a technique of historic interest.

REFERENCES

1. Acosta-Miranda AM, Will TA, Sakamoto K, et al. Stone composition differences in synchronous bilateral renal calculi. Int J Urol 2008;179(4) [supplement].
2. Lulich JP, Osborne CA. In: Bonagura J, editor. Compound uroliths: treatment and prevention. In current veterinary therapy XIII. Philadelphia: WB Saunders; 2000. p. 874–7.
3. Osborne CA. How to simplify management of complex uroliths. DVM Newsmagazine 2003;34(9):10S–3S.
4. Houston DM, Moore AEP, et al. Canine urolithiasis: a look at over 16,000 urolith submissions to the Canadian Veterinary Urolith Centre from February 1998 to April 2003. Can Vet J 2004;45:225–30.
5. Sosnar M, Bulkova T, Ruzicka M. Epidemiology of canine urolithiasis in the Czech republic from 1997 to 2002. J Small Anim Pract 2005;46:177–84.
6. Sperrin MW, Rogers K. The architecture and composition of uroliths. Br J Urol 1998;82:781–4.
7. Morshead D. Submucosal urethral calculus secondary to foxtail awn migration in a dog. J Am Vet Med Assoc 1983;182(11):1247–8.
8. Houston DM, Eaglesome H. Unusual case of foreign body-induced struvite urolithiasis in a dog. Can Vet J 1999;40:125–6.
9. Osborne CA, Bartges JW, Lulich JP, et al. Canine urolithiasis. Hand M, Thatcher C, Remillard R, editors. Small animal clinical nutrition. 4th Edition. Topeka (KS): Walsworth Publishing Co.; 2000. p. 605–88.
10. Albasan HA, Lulich JP, Osborne CA, et al. Effects of storage time and temperature on pH, specific gravity, and crystal formation in urine samples from dogs and cats. J Am Vet Med Assoc 2003;222(2):176–9.
11. Osborne CA. Minimizing pseudo-recurrent urolithiasis. DVM Newsmagazine 2005;36(5):2S–4S.

Drug-Induced Urolithiasis

Carl A. Osborne, DVM, PhD*, Jody P. Lulich, DVM, PhD,
Laurie L. Swanson, CVT, Hasan Albasan, DVM, MS, PhD

KEYWORDS

- Drug-induced crystalluria • Drug-induced uroliths • Uroliths
- Xanthine • Crystalluria • Sulfa • Fluoroquinolone

HOW DO DRUGS PROMOTE UROLITH FORMATION?

Diagnostic and therapeutic drugs may enhance urolithiasis in one or a combination of ways, including: (1) alteration of urine pH in such fashion as to create an environment that decreases or increases the solublity of some lithogenic substances; (2) alteration of glomerular filtration, tubular reabsorption, or tubular secretion of drugs or endogenous substances; (3) use of drugs that enhance promoters or impair inhibitors of urolithiasis; or (4) precipitation (eg, drugs or their metabolites) to form a portion or all of a urolith.[1,2] Likewise, toxic ingredients that are added to foods intentionally or unknowingly may produce urolithiasis (**Box 1**).

The prevalence of uroliths that contain drugs, their metabolites, or toxic ingredients in dogs, cats, and other animals is unknown. It is probable that uroliths containing drugs are often unrecognized because they are not suspected and because of limitations associated with their detection by commonly used methods of quantitative urolith analysis. For this reason, the authors recommend that the relevant drug and diet history of patients be included along with their uroliths submitted to urolith laboratories for analysis.

SULFONAMIDE ANTIMICROBICS
Risk Factors

Various types of commonly used sulfonamides are excreted primarily by glomerular filtration. Although sulfonamide crystalluria was a frequent problem associated with use of older generations of sulfonamides, newer forms of this class of drug are far less frequently associated with clinical signs attributed to sulfonamide crystalluria.

Factors that predispose to precipitation of sulfonamides, and especially their acetylated derivatives in the urinary tract, include administration of high doses of these

Veterinary Clinical Sciences Department, Minnesota Urolith Center, College of Veterinary Medicine, University of Minnesota, 1352 Boyd Avenue, St. Paul, MN 55108, USA
* Corresponding author.
E-mail address: osbor002@umn.edu (C.A. Osborne).

Vet Clin Small Anim 39 (2008) 55–63
doi:10.1016/j.cvsm.2008.09.004
0195-5616/08/$ – see front matter © 2008 Elsevier Inc. All rights reserved.

vetsmall.theclinics.com

Box 1
Some drugs and toxic food ingredients that may contribute to urolithiasis

Drugs that promote hypercalciuria

    Acidifiers

    Calcitriol

    Corticosteroids

    Furosemide

    Sodium chloride

Drugs that may decrease solubility of lithogenic substances

    Urine acidifiers

    Urine alkalinizers

Drugs that may promote hyperoxaluria

    Ascorbic acid

Drugs that may promote hyperxanthinuria

    Allopurinol

Drugs and their metabolites and food contaminants that may form portions or all of a urolith

    Urographic contrast agents

    Magnesium trisilicate melamine

    Phenazopyridine

    Fluoroquinolones

    Primodone

    Sulfonamides and their metabolites

    Tetracyclines

drugs for prolonged periods. Acid urine and highly concentrated urine are also risk factors (**Box 2**).

Epidemiology

The following data were derived from uroliths submitted to the Minnesota Urolith Center from a 10-year period beginning January 1, 1998 and ending on December 31, 2007. Using polarizing light microscopy and infrared spectroscopy to examine 373,612 canine and 77,393 feline uroliths, the authors detected sulfadiazine or its metabolites in uroliths formed by 80 dogs and 8 cats. In this series, all canine uroliths were located in the lower urinary tract, except for one ureterolith and two of unknown location. All feline uroliths were located in the lower urinary tract. Of the 80 canine patients, 49 had a history of receiving empiric treatment with a combination of sulfadiazine and trimethoprim. Six of the eight cats with sulfadiazine uroliths had a history of receiving a sulfa drug. Ling and colleagues[3] reported the occurrence of 40 sulfonamide-containing uroliths in a series of 11,000 canine uroliths. Two were observed in nephroliths.[4]

In 11 dogs and 2 cats in the authors' series, sulfadiazine or its metabolites were the only crystalline component detected in the uroliths. Ling observed sulfonamide as the

---

Box 2
Factors predisposing to precipitation of drugs in urine

Reduced volume of highly concentrated urine

Urine stasis

High rate of urinary excretion of drugs that are poorly soluble in urine

Prolonged treatment with high doses of potentially lithogenic drugs

- Sulfonamides
- Tetracyclines
- Allopurinol
- Others

---

primary component in 10 of 40 sulfa-containing specimens.[3] In 45 dogs in the authors' series, sulfadiazine or its metabolites were mixed throughout the urolith with either calcium oxalate ($n = 39$), magnesium ammonium phosphate ($n = 2$), calcium phosphate apatite ($n = 1$), magnesium ammonium phosphate mixed with calcium oxalate ($n = 1$), calcium oxalate mixed with silica ($n = 1$), or calcium oxalate mixed with calcium phosphate apatite ($n = 1$). In the authors' series, three cats had sulfadiazine or its metabolites mixed throughout the urolith with either calcium oxalate ($n = 1$), cystine ($n = 1$), or ammonium acid urate ($n = 1$). In 24 dogs in the authors' series, sulfadiazine or its metabolites were observed as a surface layer over calcium oxalate ($n = 15$), magnesium ammonium phosphate ($n = 5$), magnesium ammonium phosphate and calcium oxalate mix ($n = 2$), ammonium urate ($n = 1$), and cystine ($n = 1$). In three cats, metabolites of sulfadiazine were observed as a surface layer over magnesium ammonium phosphate ($n = 2$) and calcium oxalate ($n = 1$).

The domestic short-haired breed comprised five of eight affected cats in the authors' series. Of the eight cats with uroliths, six were neutered males and two were spayed females. The mean age of affected cats was 5 years (range = 23–144 months).

In the authors' series of 80 canine sulfa-containing uroliths, 33 different breeds of dogs were represented. Ling and colleagues[5] observed sulfa-containing uroliths in 16 breeds. In the authors' series, the mean age at the time of diagnosis was 7 years (range = 3 to 163 months). Ling and colleagues[5] reported that the mean age of dogs with sulfa residues was approximately 4 to 6 years. In the authors' series, canine sulfadiazine uroliths affected neutered (28) and intact (21) males more frequently than spayed and intact females (seven uroliths were from an unknown gender). In Ling and colleagues[5] series, 21 sulfa-containing uroliths were observed in male dogs and 19 were observed in females.

Clinical Relevance

Epidemiologic studies of case records at the Minnesota Urolith Center indicate that advancing age, male gender, and formation of acid urine are risk factors for calcium oxalate urolithiasis in dogs and cats. The authors hypothesize that the higher prevalence of sulfa-containing uroliths in older animals, especially male dogs, is confounded by unsuccessful attempts to use sulfa-containing antimicrobics to eradicate signs of lower urinary disease suspected to be caused by bacteria in dogs and cats with non-infectious metabolic uroliths (such as calcium oxalate, ammonium urate, and silica).

It is also probable that sulfadiazine is more likely to precipitate in patients with pre-existing uroliths. This phenomena is known as heterogeneous nucleation, and is somewhat analogous to the precipitation of water vapor around dust particles in the atmosphere. On the basis of available data, the authors suggest avoiding use of sulfa-diazine to empirically treat lower urinary tract signs, especially in dogs and cats known to have uroliths, known to be at increased risk for metabolic uroliths, and known to be forming acid or highly concentrated urine.

FLUOROQUINOLONES

The authors detected ciprofloxacin in multiple small (0.1 cm–0.5 cm) irregular tan-col-ored radiolucent uroliths removed from the lower urinary tract of a 6-year-old male yel-low Labrador Retriever.[6] The dog had been given multiple intermittent (7–14 day) treatments of oral ciprofloxacin (500 mg every 12 hours) over a 5-year period to treat suspected infectious bronchial disease. Since the end of December of 1997, the au-thors have detected fluoroquinolones in 15 dogs. Of the 15 uroliths retrieved from dogs, one was composed entirely of a fluoroquinolone and its metabolites. Seven were composed of a mixture of struvite and a fluoroquinolone. Four were composed of a mixture of calcium oxalate and a fluoroquinolone. Three uroliths were composed of various lithogenic salts mixed with fluoroquinolones. The mean age of this subset of uroliths was 8 years (range = 33 to 144 months). Ten different breeds were affected: seven were male, four were neutered males, two were spayed females, and one was an unspayed female (the gender of one dog was unknown). The urolith analysis form indicated that 10 of the 15 affected dogs were given a fluoroquinolone; the drug history of five dogs indicated that a fluoroquinolone was not given.

Of 77,393 uroliths retrieved from cats, a fluoroquinolone was detected in only one. This stone was retrieved from a 50-month-old neutered-male domestic short-haired cat. The stone contained a mixture of a fluoroquinolone and struvite.

Fluoroquinolones have also been reported in human nephroliths.[7]

PRIMIDONE

The authors have previously reported primidone as the only crystalline component in a urethrolith removed from an 8-year-old neutered male domestic long-haired cat.[6] According to the referring veterinarian, the cat had been treated for seizures with orally administered primidone (Mysoline) tablets (25 mg/kg given every 12 hours) during the past 7 years. Primidone crystalluria has been observed in human beings.[8]

SILICA UROLITHS

Silica uroliths have been reported in several human beings who consumed large quantities of antacids containing magnesium trisilicate to alleviate signs of peptic ulcers.[9–11]

TETRACYCLINE

Tetracycline was the primary component of multiple small yellowish, friable urocysto-liths removed from a 3-year-old male English Bulldog admitted to the University of Minnesota Veterinary Teaching Hospital.[12] The dog had been receiving large quanti-ties of orally administered tetracycline hydrochloride for at least 6 months before sur-gery in an attempt to eradicate a recalcitrant *Proteus* spp urinary tract infection. Approximately 1.5 years later, uroliths recurred in the urinary bladder, left kidney, and left ureter. The owners had apparently continued to give the dog a variety of an-tibiotics, including tetracycline, obtained from several veterinary hospitals. These uro-liths also contained tetracycline. Subsequently, studies of human patients revealed that orally administered oxytetracycline could be detected in calcium-containing uroliths.[13] The authors have not encountered any uroliths containing tetracycline since the late 1960s.

XANTHINE UROLITHS
Prevalence

Uroliths whose composition was at least 70% xanthine accounted for less than 0.1% (362 of 373,612) of all canine uroliths submitted to the Minnesota Urolith Center from 1998 to 2007. Almost all canine xanthine uroliths in the authors' series were obtained from dogs being treated with varying doses of oral allopurinol. Although xanthine has been detected as the primary mineral in feline uroliths, only one of the affected cats in the authors' series has a history of receiving allopurinol.

Age, Gender, and Breed

At the Minnesota Urolith Center, the mean age of dogs at the time of xanthine urolith retrieval was 5 years (range = 3 to 168 months). In this regard, the Cavalier King Charles Spaniel is an exception inasmuch that naturally occurring xanthine uroliths have been recognized when these dogs were less than 1 year of age.[14]

Male dogs (86%) were affected more often than females (9%) in the authors' series (5% were of unknown gender). Of these dogs, 190 were castrated males (53%), 122 were intact males (34%), 23 were spayed females (6%), 11 were nonspayed females (3%), and 16 were of unknown gender (4%). With the apparent exception of Cavalier King Charles spaniels (six dogs in the series), the predominance of allopurinol-induced xanthine uroliths in males has also been observed by others.[3,13] In a report of 38 xanthine-containing uroliths, 36 occurred in males and 2 occurred in females.[3]

At the authors' center, 40 different breeds were affected, including Dalmatians (50%), mixed breed (12%), English Bulldogs (4%), Miniature Schnauzers (4%), German Shepherds (2%), Boxers (2%), and Cavalier King Charles Spaniels (2%). Similar observations have been made by others.[15] In a recent report, of 38 xanthine-containing uroliths, 30 were found in Dalmatians, 2 were found in Miniature or Toy Poodles, and one was retrieved from a Shih Tzu. The affected breeds for five xanthine specimens was apparently unknown. Of the 362 uroliths composed of xanthine in the authors' series, 316 dogs were given allopurinol, 10 were given fluoroquinolones, and 2 received sulfadiazine (34 uroliths were submitted without a drug history).

Mineral Composition, Location, and Number

Quantitative analyses of canine xanthine uroliths submitted to the authors' center have revealed that most are pure, but a few contain other minerals, especially ammonium urate or sodium and calcium salts of uric acid. This is expected because allopurinol is commonly used to treat and prevent uroliths containing these salts. However, layers of xanthine were also observed surrounding uroliths composed of calcium oxalate, cystine, or struvite. The center of one urolith removed from a 6-year-old male Chihuahua was composed of a mixture of calcium oxalate (30%) and calcium phosphate (70%), and was surrounded by a shell containing xanthine (70%) and sulfadiazine (30%).

Pure xanthine urocystoliths were usually ovoid and smooth. Except for their yellow to yellow-brown color (xanthine is the Latin word for "yellow"), they resembled ammonium urate uroliths (**Fig. 1**). They varied in diameter from 0.5 mm to approximately 1 cm. Uroliths containing xanthine were more commonly removed from the lower urinary tract of dogs (94%) than the upper urinary tract (6%). The number of xanthine-containing uroliths in each patient varied from 1 to more than 100.

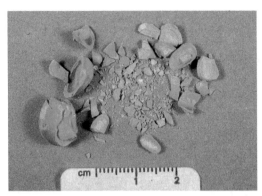

Fig. 1. Urocystoliths removed from a 3-year-old spayed Yorkshire terrier being treated for ammonium urate urolithiasis with orally administered allopurinol. The inner portion of the sectioned urolith is omposed of ammonium urate. The outer layers of the sectioned stone are composed of xanthine.

Etiopathogenesis

Xanthine is a product of purine metabolism and is converted to uric acid by the enzyme xanthine oxidase (**Fig. 2**). Hereditary xanthinuria is a disorder characterized by a deficiency of xanthine oxidase. As a consequence, abnormal quantities of xanthine are excreted in urine as a major end-product of purine metabolism. Because xanthine is the least soluble of the purines excreted in urine, xanthinuria may be associated with formation of uroliths. Naturally occurring xanthinuria was recognized in a family of Cavalier King Charles Spaniels in the Netherlands. An autosomal recessive mode inheritance was postulated.[13]

The authors have observed xanthine in 171 of 77,393 feline urolith specimens submitted to the Minnesota Urolith Center from 1998 to 2007. Only one of the cats had been treated with allopurinol. This feline xanthine series comprised 11 different breeds (including domestic short hair, 70%; domestic long hair, 17%; domestic medium hair, 5%; and Siamese, 2%). The mean age of affected cats was 3 years (range = 3 –176

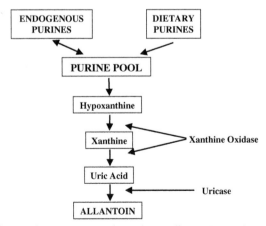

Fig. 2. Diagram of normal canine purine degradation illustrating action of xanthine oxidase to convert xanthine to uric acid and allantoin.

months). The genders were 94 (55%) male neutered, 17 (10%) nonneutered males, 57 (33%) spayed females, and 2 (1%) nonspayed females. The gender of one cat was not reported. Thirty-seven cats had recurrent urolithiasis.

Most xanthine uroliths in dogs form secondary to therapy with allopurinol.[15,16] Allopurinol rapidly binds to and inhibits the action of xanthine oxidase, thereby decreasing conversion of hypoxanthine to xanthine and xanthine to uric acid. The result is a reduction of serum and urine concentrations of uric acid, with an increase in serum and urine concentrations of xanthine. Administration of allopurinol at high doses, especially with concurrent consumption of high-purine diets, has resulted in formation of xanthine uroliths.[15,16]

Diagnosis

Urinalysis
Xanthine crystals in urine sediment cannot be distinguished from many forms of ammonium urate or amorphous urates (**Figs. 3** and **4**).[17] Xanthine crystals are usually brown or yellow-brown and may form spherules of varying size.

Detection of xanthinuria
Xanthinuria may be detected by high-pressure liquid chromatography. In one study, xanthine concentrations in urine obtained from beagle dogs could be reproducibly measured in undiluted or diluted samples preserved by freezing for up to 12 weeks.[18,19] However, reliable measurements of uric acid in frozen urine required dilution of the sample (1 part urine to 20 parts deionized water).

Radiography and ultrasonography
The size of xanthine uroliths varied from that just detectable by the unaided eye to approximately 1 cm. The radiodensity of xanthine uroliths compared with soft tissue is similar to that of ammonium urate uroliths, but somewhat less than struvite and silica uroliths, and substantially less than calcium oxalate and calcium phosphate uroliths. Some xanthine uroliths were radiolucent.

Double-contrast cystography is more sensitive in detecting small xanthine urocystoliths than survey radiography and most techniques of ultrasonography. Xanthine uroliths appear as radiolucent uroliths when surrounded by, but not completely submerged in, radiopaque contrast medium. Survey radiography may be insensitive in detecting xanthine urethroliths. Positive contrast urography may be required to detect and localize xanthine uroliths that have passed into the urethral lumen.

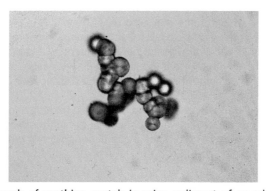

Fig. 3. Photomicrograh of xanthine crystals in urine sediment of an adult female beagle given allopurinol orally and a diet unrestricted in purine precursors.

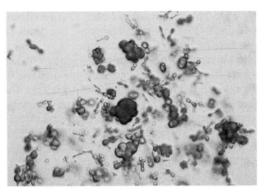

Fig. 4. Photomicrograh of ammonium urate crystals in urine sediment of a 10-year-old neutered male Dalmatian. Compare with the xanthine crystals in **Fig. 3** (unstained, 40x original magnification).

Although uroliths can be detected by ultrasonography, this method does not provide information about the degree of their radiodensity or shape. Evaluation of the density and shape of uroliths often provides useful information in predicting their mineral type.

Quantitative urolith analysis

Quantitative analysis of uroliths provides a definitive diagnosis of xanthine urolithiasis. Uroliths may be collected with a tropical fish net during the voiding phase of micturition, by aspiration through a urinary catheter, or by voiding urohydropropulsion. Polarizing light microscopy is an insensitive method to detect xanthine as a component of uroliths. Infrared spectroscopy can be used to confirm that uroliths contain xanthine.

Prevention and Treatment

The magnitude of allopurinol induced xanthinuria is influenced by several variables including: (1) the dosage of allopurinol, (2) the quantity of purine precursors in the diet, (3) the rate of production of endogenous purine precursors, (4) the rate and completeness of endogenous and exogenous degradation and, (5) the status of hepatic function and its influence on the pharmacokinetics of allopurinol and its metabolites.

To minimize the likelihood of inducing xanthine urolith formation, simultaneous consumption of purine-rich or purine-supplemented diets should be avoided. Feeding high-moisture canned diets to reduce urine concentration is highly recommended. Minimizing formation of acid urine may also be of benefit. It is probable that a dog who has developed xanthine uroliths as a result of treating urate uroliths, and consuming a diet that has not been evaluated for purine content, would benefit from discontinuing allopurinol therapy (or at least reducing the daily dosage), and given a trial of therapy with a purine-restricted, high-moisture nonacidifying diet (such as Prescription Diet canine u/d canned: Hill's Pet Nutrition).

To minimize xanthine urolith recurrence in cats, avoid treating affected patients with allopurinol. Feeding a reduced-purine, nonacidifying, high-moisture diet may be of benefit in reducing the rate of recurrence of xanthine uroliths in cats.

REFERENCES

1. Koneman EW, Schessler J. Unusual urinary crystals. Technical Bulletin of the Registry of Medical Technologists 1965;35:144.

2. Jones HM, Schrader WA. Ampicillin crystalluria. Am J Clin Path 1972;58:220–3.
3. Ling GV, Franti CE, Ruby AL, et al. Urolithiasis in dogs I: mineral prevalence and interrelations of mineral composition, age, and sex. Am J Vet Res 1998;59:624–9.
4. Ling GV, Ruby AL, Johnson DL, et al. Renal calculi in dogs and cats: prevalence, mineral type, breed, age, and gender interrelationships (1981–1993). J Vet Intern Med 1998;12:11–21.
5. Ling GV, Franti CE, Ruby AL, et al. Urolithiasis in dogs II: breed prevalence, and interrelations of breed, sex, age, and mineral composition. Am J Vet Res 1998;59: 630–42.
6. Osborne CA, Lulich JP, Bartges JW, et al. Drug induced urolithiasis. Vet Clin North Am 1999;28(1):251–66.
7. Rince C, Daudon M, Moesch C, et al. Identification of flumequine in a urinary calculus. J Clin Chem Clin Biochem. 1987;25:313–4.
8. Bailey DN, Jatlow PL. Chemical analysis of massive crystalluria following primidone overdose. Am J Clin Path 1972;58:583–9.
9. Farber JH, Raifer J. Silicate urolithiasis. J Urol 1984;132:739–40.
10. Levison DA, Crocker PR, Banim S, et al. Silica stones in the urinary bladder. Lancet 1982;1:704–5.
11. Medina JA, Sanchidrian JR, Cifuentes Delatte L. Silica in urinary calculi. In: Smith LH, Robertson WG, Finlayson B, editors. Urolithiasis: clinical and basic research. New York: Plenum Press; 1981. p. 923–6.
12. Osborne CA, Oldroyd NO, Clinton CW. Etipopathogenesis of uncommon canine uroliths. Xanthine, drugs, and drug metabolites. Vet Clin North Am Small Anim Pract 1986;16:217–25 (Article provides additional information about drugs and drug metabolites in uroliths).
13. Mulvaney WP, Beck CW, Qureshi MA. Occurrence of tetracycline in urinary calculi. J Urol 1965;94:187–91.
14. van Zuilen CD, Nickel RF, Van Dijk TH, et al. Xanthinuria in a family of Cavalier King Charles spaniels. Vet Q 1997;19:172–4.
15. Ling GV, Ruby AL, Harrold DR, et al. Xanthine-containing urinary calculi in dogs given allopurinol. J Am Vet Med Assoc 1991;198:1935–40.
16. Bartges JW, Osborne CA, Felice LJ. Canine xanthine uroliths: risk factor management. In: Kirk RW, Bonagura JD, editors. Current veterinary therapy XI. Philadelphia: WB Saunders Co; 1992. p. 900–5.
17. Osborne CA, Stevens JB, Luilich JP, et al. A clinician's analysis of urinalysis. In: Osborne CA, Finco DR, editors. Canine and feline nephrology and urology. Baltimore, Maryland: Williams & Wilkins; 1995. p. 136–205.
18. Bartges JW, Osborne CA, Felice LJ, et al. Effects of time and dilution on concentration of xanthine in frozen urine and plasma of dogs. Am J Vet Res 1997;58: 118–20.
19. Holmes EW, Wyngaarden JB. Hereditary xanthinuria. In: Scriver CR, Beaudet AL, Sly WL, editors. 6th edition, The Metabolic Basis of Inherited Disease. vol. I. New York: McGraw Hill; 1989. p. 1085–94.

Quantitative Analysis of 4468 Uroliths Retrieved from Farm Animals, Exotic Species, and Wildlife Submitted to the Minnesota Urolith Center: 1981 to 2007

Carl A. Osborne, DVM, PhD[a], Hasan Albasan, DVM, MS, PhD[a],
Jody P. Lulich, DVM, PhD[a], Eugene Nwaokorie, DVM[b], Lori A. Koehler, CVT[a],
Lisa K. Ulrich, CVT[a]

KEYWORDS

- Exotic • Zoo • Wildlife • Uroliths • Calculi
- Quantitative analysis

Knowledge of the mineral composition of uroliths in various species of animals can often help veterinarians predict the mineral composition of stones in vivo. This information is important because dissolution of existing uroliths, or minimizing further growth of uroliths in situ, is dependent on knowledge of the mineral composition of uroliths.

With this objective in mind, this report summarizes the results of quantitative mineral analysis of uroliths retrieved from 4468 farm animals, wildlife, and so-called "exotic" species of animals and sent to the Minnesota Urolith Center by various individuals living primarily in North America, Eastern Europe, Australia, New Zealand, and Asia. We have reported the methods we used to identify and classify various minerals found in these uroliths.[1] The information provided in this report summarizes the most extensive database about uroliths from animals other than domesticated dogs and domesticated cats that we could identify in the literature.

Supported in part by an educational grant from Hill's Pet Nutrition, Topeka, Kansas.
[a] Veterinary Clinical Sciences Department, Minnesota Urolith Center, College of Veterinary Medicine, University of Minnesota, 1352 Boyd Avenue, St. Paul, MN 55108, USA
[b] Minnesota Urolith Center, College of Veterinary Medicine, University of Minnesota, 1352 Boyd Avenue, St. Paul, MN 55108, USA
E-mail address: osbor002@umn.edu (C.A. Osborne).

We have also included selected reports of uroliths in the English literature related to specific stones that we have evaluated (**Appendix 1**). We did not include reports of uroliths whose composition was not described, or reports of uroliths evaluated by insensitive qualitative techniques.

We encourage our colleagues to continue to send us uroliths retrieved from farm animals, exotic species, and wildlife for evaluation by quantitative techniques. Because of the strong support of an educational grant from Hill's Pet Nutrition, we are able to provide this service without a monetary fee. However, to gain insights into the epidemiology of urolithiasis, we ask that each submission be accompanied by a one page urolith analysis request form. This form can be found at our Web site: www.cvm.umn.edu. Click on the link to department and centers to find Minnesota Urolith Center, and follow the menu to the request form. The details are available under the icon labeled "How to submit samples." For colleagues residing outside the borders of the United States, packaging instructions for noninfectious clinical samples may be found at: http://www.usps.com/, US Postal Service Packaging Instruction 6C. Alternatively, contact your preferred shipper for instructions about complying with International Air Transportion Association Regulation 3.6.2.2.3.6. We comply with all federal and state regulations regarding handling and shipment of samples that are a potential source of diseases that are communicable to animals and humans. Information on acceptable species for USA importation and documentation necessary for the United States Department of Agriculture (USDA) customs inspection can be found under guidelines 1102, 1103, and 1104 at: www.aphis.usda.gov/.

Appendix 1
Quantitative analysis of 4468 uroliths retrieved from farm animals, exotic species, and wildlife sent to the Minnesota Urolith Center: 1981–2007

Animals	No. (%)
Carnivore	
Bobcat uroliths (n=2)	
Struvite	2 (100)
Bush dog uroliths (n=2)	
Struvite	1 (50)
Purines	1 (50)
Cape hunting dog uroliths (n=1)	
Calcium phosphate	1 (100)
Caracal (Persian lynx) uroliths (n=3)	
Calcium oxalate	2 (66.7)
Miscellaneous	(33.3)
Cheetah uroliths[2] (n=2)	
Calcium phosphate	1 (50)
Purines	1 (50)
Cougar uroliths (n=1)	
Calcium phosphate	1 (100)
Cusimanse (Dark mongoose) uroliths (n=3)	
Calcium oxalate	2 (66.7)
Compound	1 (33.3)

Ferret uroliths[a][3,4] (n=409)	
Struvite	273 (66.8)
Cystine	61 (14.9)
Calcium oxalate	43 (10.5)
Purines	8 (2.0)
Matrix	6 (1.5)
Compound	4 (1.0)
Mixed	4 (1.0)
Other	4 (1.0)
Calcium phosphate	3 (0.7)
Silica	1 (0.2)
Calcium carbonate	1 (0.2)
Magnesium hydrogen phosphate	1 (0.2)
Fox uroliths[b] (n=27)	
Struvite	21 (77.8)
Cystine	3 (11.1)
Calcium oxalate	1 (3.7)
Calcium phosphate	1 (3.7)
Compound	1 (3.7)
Leopard uroliths[c] (n=14)	
Struvite	5 (35.7)
Calcium oxalate	1 (7.1)
Calcium phosphate	3 (21.4)
Mixed	3 (21.4)
Compound	1 (7.1)
Miscellaneous	1 (7.1)
Lion uroliths[5,6] (n=6)	
Calcium oxalate	4 (66.66)
Struvite	1 (16.66)
Mixed	1 (16.66)
Lynx uroliths[7] (n=2)	
Calcium oxalate	1 (50)
Silica	1 (50)
Mink uroliths[d] (n=22)	
Struvite	22 (100)
Mongoose uroliths (n=4)	
Calcium phosphate	2 (50)
Mixed	2 (50)
Otter uroliths[e][8–11] (n=108)	
Calcium oxalate	60 (55.6)
Compound	29 (26.9)
Purines	9 (8.33)
Mixed	6 (5.6)
Calcium carbonate	2 (1.9)
Struvite	2 (1.9)

(continued on next page)

Appendix 1 *(continued)*	
Animals	**No. (%)**
Raccoon uroliths[12] (n=21)	
Purines	17 (80.9)
Compound	2 (9.5)
Calcium oxalate	1 (4.8)
Mixed	1 (4.8)
Tiger uroliths[f] (n=3)	
Struvite	2 (66.7)
Miscellaneous	1 (33.3)
Wolf uroliths[g13] (n=39)	
Cystine	30 (76.9)
Struvite	4 (10.3)
Mixed	2 (5.1)
Calcium oxalate	1 (2.6)
Compound	1 (2.6)
Other	1 (2.6)
Ruminant	
Bison uroliths (n=2)	
Calcium oxalate	2 (100)
Bongo (large, forest-dwelling antelope) uroliths (n=2)	
Calcium oxalate	2 (100)
Bovine (domestic) uroliths[14–24] (n=217)	
Struvite	73 (33.6)
Silica	43 (19.8)
Magnesium calcium phosphate	8 (3.7)
Magnesium calcium phosphate carbonate	28 (12.9)
Compound	17 (7.8)
Calcium phosphate	17 (7.8)
Mixed	14 (6.5)
Calcium carbonate	8 (3.7)
Calcium oxalate	4 (1.8)
Purines	2 (0.9)
Matrix	2 (0.9)
Other	1 (0.5)
Camel uroliths[25] (n=5)	
Silica	4 (80)
Purines	1 (20)
Caprine (domestic) uroliths[26–32] (n=526)	
Calcium carbonate	224 (42.6)
Magnesium calcium phosphate carbonate	101 (19.2)
Silica	76 (14.5)
Compound	34 (6.5)
Magnesium calcium phosphate	24 (4.6)
Struvite	19 (3.6)

Mixed	21 (4)
Calcium phosphate	16 (3)
Calcium oxalate	4 (0.8)
Other	4 (0.8)
Matrix	2 (0.4)
Purines	1 (0.1)
Caribou (reindeer-like animal) uroliths (n=3)	
Calcium oxalate	3 (100)
Deer uroliths[33] (n=12)	
Struvite	3 (25)
Magnesium calcium phosphate	2 (16.7)
Magnesium calcium phosphate carbonate	2 (16.7)
Mixed	2 (16.7)
Calcium phosphate	1 (8.3)
Calcium carbonate	1 (8.3)
Miscelleneous	1 (8.3)
Duiker (small antelope) uroliths (n=4)	
Struvite	1 (25)
Purines	1 (25)
Magnesium calcium phosphate carbonate	1 (25)
Mixed	1 (25)
Gazelle (African antelope) uroliths (n=1)	
Purines	1 (100)
Gemsbok (large African antelope) uroliths (n=1)	
Calcium phosphate	1 (100)
Giraffe uroliths[34] (n=12)	
Magnesium calcium phosphate carbonate	4 (33.3)
Magnesium calcium phosphate	3 (25)
Mixed	3 (25)
Struvite	1 (8.3)
Other	1 (8.3)
Greater Kudu (Woodland antelope) uroliths (n=5)	
Other	2 (40)
Magnesium calcium phosphate	1 (20)
Calcium phosphate	1 (20)
Miscellaneous	1 (20)
Llama uroliths[35,36] (n=24)	
Silica	18 (75)
Struvite	2 (8.3)
Calcium phosphate	1 (4.2)
Purines	1 (4.2)
Magnesium calcium phosphate carbonate	1 (4.2)
Calcium carbonate	1 (4.2)
Moose uroliths (n=2)	
Calcium carbonate	2 (100)

(continued on next page)

Appendix 1 *(continued)*	
Animals	**No. (%)**
Mouflon (wild mountain sheep) uroliths (n=5)	
Calcium phosphate	2 (40)
Struvite	1 (20)
Magnesium calcium phosphate	1 (20)
Mixed	1 (20)
Muntjac (type of deer) uroliths (n=1)	
Calcium phosphate	1 (100)
Ovine (domestic) uroliths[21,22,29,31,37–39] (n=111)	
Calcium carbonate	33 (29.7)
Magnesium calcium phosphate carbonate	22 (19.8)
Struvite	16 (14.4)
Calcium phosphate	14 (12.6)
Silica	12 (10.8)
Mixed	7 (6.3)
Matrix	3 (2.7)
Compound	2 (1.8)
Calcium oxalate	1 (0.9)
Other	1 (0.9)
Tahr (goat-like animal) uroliths (n=4)	
Purines	3 (75)
Calcium phosphate	1 (25)
Wildebeest uroliths (n=4)	
Calcium carbonate	3 (75)
Purines	1 (25)
Equine	
Equine (domestic) uroliths[40–49] (n=256)	
Calcium carbonate	243 (94.9)
Compound	4 (1.6)
Struvite	3 (1.2)
Calcium oxalate monohydrate	2 (0.8)
Magnesium calcium phosphate carbonate	1 (0.4)
Mixed	1 (0.4)
Matrix	1 (0.4)
Other	1 (0.4)
Porcine	
Peccary (pig-like hoofed mammal) uroliths (n=1)	
Compound	1 (100)
Porcine (domestic) uroliths[50–55] (n=95)	
Calcium phosphate	33 (34.7)
Struvite	18 (18.9)
Mixed	13 (13.7)
Magnesium calcium phosphate carbonate	9 (9.5)
Compound	9 (9.5)

Magnesium calcium phosphate	3 (3.2)
Calcium carbonate	3 (3.2)
Silica	3 (3.2)
Calcium oxalate	2 (2.1)
Purines	1 (1.1)
Other	1 (1.1)
Rodent	
Rabbit (domestic) uroliths[56–61] (n=1011)	
Calcium carbonate	702 (69.4)
Compound	232 (23)
Mixed	33 (3.3)
Calcium phosphate	14 (1.4)
Magnesium calcium phosphate carbonate	11 (1.1)
Calcium oxalate	9 (0.9)
Silica	4 (0.4)
Magnesium calcium phosphate	3 (0.3)
Struvite	2 (0.2)
Matrix	1 (<0.01)
Capybara (large South American rodent) uroliths (n=2)	
Calcium carbonate	2 (100)
Chinchilla uroliths[62,63] (n=73)	
Calcium carbonate	64 (87.7)
Miscellaneous	5 (6.8)
Compound	4 (5.5)
Groundhog uroliths (n=1)	
Struvite	1 (100)
Guinea pig uroliths[64–68] (n=948)	
Calcium carbonate	878 (92.6)
Compound	27 (2.8)
Mixed	15 (1.6)
Calcium phosphate	10 (1.1)
Matrix	9 (1.0)
Calcium oxalate	4 (0.4)
Magnesium calcium phosphate	2 (0.2)
Other	2 (0.2)
Struvite	1 (0.1)
Hamster uroliths (n=14)	
Calcium phosphate	4 (28.6)
Compound	4 (28.6)
Calcium oxalate	3 (21.4)
Struvite	2 (14.3)
Mixed	1 (7.1)
Mice uroliths[69,70] (n=39)	
Struvite	37 (94.9)
Matrix	2 (5.1)

(continued on next page)

Appendix 1 (continued)	
Animals	**No. (%)**
Porcupine uroliths (n=3)	
Calcium phosphate	1 (33 3)
Compound	1 (33.3)
Matrix	1 (33.3)
Rat uroliths[71–77] (n=51)	
Struvite	41 (80.4)
Calcium phosphate	3 (5.9)
Calcium carbonate	2 (3.9)
Other	2 (3.9)
Mixed	1 (2)
Magnesium hydrogen phosphate	1 (2)
Magnesium calcium phosphate carbonate	1 (2)
Squirrel uroliths (n=2)	
Purine	1 (50)
Compound	1 (50)
Marsupial	
Kangaroo uroliths[78,79] (n=15)	
Calcium carbonate	8 (71.9)
Calcium oxalate	3 (20)
Compound	2 (13.3)
Silica	1 (6.7)
Purines	1 (6.7)
Opossum uroliths (n=8)	
Struvite	7 (87.5)
Mixed	1 (12.5)
Wallaby uroliths (n=7)	
Calcium carbonate	6 (85.7)
Compound	1 (14.3)
Wombat uroliths[h] (n=1)	
Calcium oxalate	1 (100)
Cetacea	
Dolphin uroliths[80] (n=13)	
Purines	11 (84.6)
Calcium phosphate carbonate	1 (7.7)
Struvite	1 (7.7)
Harbor porpoise uroliths (n=1)	
Struvite	1 (100)
Whale uroliths[81] (n=2)	
Calcium phosphate	1 (50)
Purines	1 (50)
Fish	
Angel fish uroliths (n=2)	
Calcium phosphate	2 (100)

Lion fish uroliths[i] (n=3)	
Calcium phosphate carbonate	3 (100)
Northern kingfish uroliths[j] (n=1)	
Calcium hydrogen phosphate dehydrate	1 (100)
Porkfish uroliths[k] (n=1)	
Calcium phosphate	1 (100)
Rainbow trout uroliths (n=1)	
Calcium phosphate carbonate	1 (100)
Sand tiger shark uroliths (n=1)	
Calcium phosphate carbonate	1 (100)
Primate	
Ape and monkey uroliths[82–84] (n=42)	
Calcium carbonate	26 (62)
Calcium oxalate	7 (16.6)
Struvite	2 (4.7)
Cystine	2 (4.7)
Calcium phosphate	4 (9.5)
Matrix	1 (2.3)
Reptile	
Gecko uroliths (n=2)	
Other	1 (50)
Purines	1 (50)
Iguana uroliths[85] (n=140)	
Purines	136 (97.1)
Mixed	3 (2.1)
Compound	1 (0.7)
Lizard uroliths (n=26)	
Purines	24 (92.3)
Calcium carbonate	1 (3.8)
Compound	1 (3.8)
Tortoise uroliths (n=66)	
Purines	62 (93.9)
Calcium carbonate	2 (3.0)
Mixed	2 (3.0)
Turtle uroliths[86] (n=12)	
Purines	7 (58.3)
Calcium phosphate	2 (16.7)
Compound	2 (16.7)
Mixed	1 (8.3)
Other	
Elephant uroliths (n=3)	
Calcium carbonate	2 (66.6)
Calcium phosphate	1 (33.3)
Harbor seal uroliths[187] (n=3)	
Purines	3 (100)

(continued on next page)

Appendix 1 (continued)	
Animals	**No. (%)**
Hippopotamus uroliths (n=2)	
Calcium oxalate	2 (100)
Shrew uroliths (n=2)	
Struvite	1 (50)
Calcium oxalate	1 (50)
Sloth uroliths (n=7)	
Struvite	3 (42.9)
Compound	2 (28.6)
Magnesium phosphate	1 (14.3)
Mixed	1 (14.3)
Tapir uroliths[m] (n=1)	
Calcium carbonate	1 (100)
Total	**4468**

[a] Studies are in progress to determine if naturally occurring sterile-struvite uroliths can be safely dissolved by formulating an urine-acidfying magnesium-restricted diet.

[b] Information regarding the status of urinary tract infections is unknown. Therefore, we cannot determine if the struvite uroliths were induced by urease producing microbes or if the struvite formed in sterile urine.

[c] Please see comments for fox uroliths.

[d] Struvite uroliths in mink are usually the result of urinary tract infections with urease-producing microbes.

[e] Calcium oxalate uroliths are very common in captive Asian small clawed otters. Uroliths composed of salts of uric acid have been observed in American river otters and Eurasian otters.

[f] Please see comments for fox uroliths.

[g] We have observed cystine uroliths in several grey wolves living in northern Minnesota.

[h] Australian marsupials are short-legged muscular quadrupeds, approximately 39 inches in length with a very short tail.

[i] Otherwise known as turkey fish or dragon fish. Lionfish are venomous and are noted for their extremely long and separated spines. They usually have a striped appearance: red, brown, orange, yellow, black, maroon, or white.

[j] Kingfish is the common name of a number of different species of fish, including the king mackerel, the cero, the northern kingfish (also called northern king whiting), and the southern kingfish (southern king whiting). The northern kingfish is a bottom-dwelling fish that feeds on shrimp, small fish, and crabs. It grows to a length of 18 inches, and is found in coastal waters from Massachusetts to Yucatán.

[k] Also known as grunts. A member of the grunt family, the porkfish can produce a peculiar grunting sound by rubbing together the teeth in its throat. They have a "smiling" expression when their mouths are closed. When open, their mouths show a bright red lining, which they often display to each other in territorial contests. Grunts are a group of small to midsize bass-like fishes that have deep, compressed, oval-shaped bodies.

[l] Elephant seals and sea lions (or sea elephants) are a true seal of the genus Mirounga. They are the largest of the fin-footed mammals, or pinnipeds, exceeding the walrus in size. The eared seals (or otariids) are marine mammals in the family Otariidae, one of three groupings of Pinnipeds. They comprise 16 species in seven genera commonly known either as sea lions or fur seals, distinct from true seals (phocids) and walruses (odobenids).[88]

[m] Tapirs (pronounced "taper" or "ta-pier") are large browsing mammals, roughly pig-like in shape, with short prehensile snouts.

REFERENCES

1. Ulrich LK, Bird KA, Koehler LA, et al. Urolith analysis: submission, methods, and interpretation. Vet Clin North Am Small Anim Pract 1996;339–415.
2. Weber WJ, Raphael BL, Boothe HW. Struvite uroliths in a cheetah. JAVMA 1984; 185:1389–90.
3. Dutton MA. Treatment of cystine bladder urolith in a ferret (*Mustela putorius furo*). Exotic Pet Practice 1996;1:7.
4. Palmore WP, Bartos KD. Food intake and struvite crystalluria in ferrets. Vet Res Commun 1987;11:519–26.
5. Corpa JM, Marin S, Bolea R, et al. Urolithiasis in two lions. Vet Rec 2003;153: 786–7.
6. Fletcher KC. Obstructive uropathy in a lion. Feline Practice 1980;10:45–8.
7. Jackson OF, Jones DM. Cystine calculi in a caracal lynx. J Comp Pathol 1979;89: 39–42.
8. Calle PP, Robinson PT. Glucosuria associated with renal calculi in Asian small-clawed otters. JAVMA 1985;187:1149–53.
9. Grove RA, Bildfell R, Charles JH, et al. Bilateral uric acid nephrolithiasis and ureteral hypertrophy in a free-ranging river otter (*Lontra Canadensis*). J Wildl Dis 2003;39:914–7.
10. Petrini KR, Lulich JP, Treschel L, et al. Evaluation of urinary and serum metabolites in Asian small-clawed otters (*Aonyx cinerea*) with calcium oxalate urolithiasis. J Zoo Wildl Med 1999;30(1):54–63.
11. Weber H, Steffes HJ, Steinlechner, et al. Ammonium urate lithiasis: specific occurrence in Eurasian otters, Lutra lutra. In: Proceedings of the 9th International Symposium on Urolithiasis 2000;836–8.
12. Page CD, Probst CW. Ammonium urate renal calculus in a raccoon. J Am Vet Med Assoc 1981;179:1259–61 [Describes ammonium urate nephrolith in a raccoon].
13. Bush M, Bovee KC. Cystinuria in a maned wolf. J Am Vet Med Assoc 1978;173: 1159–62.
14. Braun U, Nuss K, Sydler T, et al. Ultrasonographic findings in three cows with ureteral obstruction due to urolithiasis. Vet Rec 2006;159:750–2.
15. Floyd JG. Urolithiasis in food animals. In: Howard JL, Smith RA, editors. Current veterinary therapy. Food animal practice. 4th edition. Philadelphia: W.B. Saunders Co; 1999. p. 621–4.
16. Gasthuys F, Steenhaut M, De Moor A, et al. Surgical treatment of urethral obstruction due to urolithiasis in male cattle: a review of 85 cases. Vet Rec 1993;133: 522–6.
17. Hawkins WW. Experimental production and control of urolithiasis. J Am Vet Med Assoc 1965;147:1321–3.
18. Larson BL. Identifying, treating, and preventing bovine urolithiasis. Vet Med 1996; 91:366–72.
19. McIntosh GH. Urolithiasis in animals. Aust Vet J 1978;54:267–71.
20. McIntosh GH, Pulsford MF, Spencer WG, et al. A study of urolithiasis in grazing ruminants in south Australia. Aust Vet J 1974;50:345–50.
21. Nottle MC. Composition of some urinary calculi of ruminants in western Australia. Res Vet Sci 1976;21:309–13.

22. Romanowski RD. Biochemistry of urolith formation. J Am Vet Med Assoc 1965; 147:1324–5.
23. Sutor DJ, Wooley SE. Animal calculi: an X-Ray diffraction study of their crystalline composition. Res Vet Sci 1970;11:299–301.
24. Waltner-Toewsand D, Meadows DH. Urolithiasis in a herd of beef cattle associated with oxalate ingestion. Can Vet J 1980;21:61–2.
25. Gutierrez C, Corbera JA, Doreste F, et al. Silica urolithiasis in the dromedary camel in a subtropical climate. J Res Commun 2002;26:437–42.
26. Clark P, Swenson CL, Osborne CA, et al. Calcium oxalate crystalluria in a goat. J Am Vet Med Assoc 1999;215:77–8.
27. Ewoldt JM, Anderson DE, Miesner MD, et al. Short- and long-term outcome and factors predicting survival after surgical tube cystostomy for treatment of obstructive urolithiasis in small ruminants. Vet Surg 2006;35:417–22.
28. Halland SK, House JK, George LW. Urethroscopy and laser lithotripsy for the diagnosis and treatment of obstructive urolithiasis in goats and pot-bellied pigs. J Am Vet Med Assoc 2002;220:1831–4.
29. Kimberling CV, Arnold KS. Disease of the urinary system of sheep and goats. Vet Clin North Am Large Anim Pract 1983;5:637–55.
30. McIntosh GH. Urolithiasis in animals. Aust Vet J 1978;54:267–71.
31. Rakestraw PC, Fubini SL, Gilbert RO, et al. Tube cystostomy for treatment of obstructive urolithiasis in small ruminants. Vet Surg 1995;24:498–505.
32. Streeter RN, Washburn KE, McCauley CT. Percutaneous tube cystostomy and vesicular irrigation for treatment of obstructive urolithiasis in a goat. J Am Vet Med Assoc 2002;221:546–9.
33. Reynolds RN. Urolithiasis in a wild red deer (Cervus elaphus) population. N Z Vet J 1982;30:25–6.
34. Wolfe BA, Sladky KK, Loomis MR. Obstructive urolithiasis in a reticulated giraffe (Giraffa camelopardalis reticulate). Vet Rec 2000;146:260–1.
35. Kingston JK, Staempfli HR. Silica urolithiasis in a male llama. Can Vet J 1995;36: 767–8.
36. Kock MD, Fowler ME. Urolithiasis in a three-month-old llama. J Am Vet Med Assoc 1982;181:1411.
37. Ewoldt JM, Anderson DE, Miesner MD, et al. Short- and long-term outcome and factors predicting survival after surgical tube cystostomy for treatment of obstructive urolithiasis in small ruminants. Vet Surg 2006;35:417–22.
38. McIntosh GH. Urolithiasis in animals. Aust Vet J 1978;54:267–71.
39. Stewart SR, Emerick RJ, Pritchard RH. Effects of dietary ammonium chloride and variations in calcium to phosphorus ratio on silica urolithiasis in sheep. J Anim Sci 1991;69:2225–9.
40. DeBowes MR, Nyrop KA. Cystic calculi in the horse. Comp Cont Edu 1984;6: S268–73.
41. Diaz-Espineira M, Escolar E, Bellanato J, et al. Crystalline composition of equine urinary sabulous deposits. Scanning Microsc 1995;9:1071–9.
42. Diaz-Espineira M, Escolar E, Bellanato J, et al. Minor constituents of sabulous material in equine urine. Res Vet Sci 1996;60:238–42.
43. Diaz-Espineira M, Escolar E, Bellanato J, et al. Structure and composition of equine uroliths. J Equine Vet Sci 1995;15:27–34.
44. Diaz-Espineira M, Nellanato J, De La Fuente MA. Infrared and atomic spectrometry analysis of the mineral composition of a series of equine sabulous material and urinary calculi. Res Vet Sci 1997;63:93–5.

45. Ehnen SJ, Divers TJ, Gillette D, et al. Obstructive nephrolithiasis and ureterolithiasis associated with chronic renal failure in horses: eight cases (1981–1987). J Am Vet Med Assoc 1990;97:249–53.
46. Holt PE, Pearson H. Urolithiasis in the horse—a review of 13 cases. Equine Vet J 1984;16:31–4.
47. Laverty S, Pascoe JR, Ling GV, et al. Urolithiasis in 68 horses. Vet Surg 1992;21: 56–62.
48. McIntosh GH. Urolithiasis in animals. Aust Vet J 1978;54:267–71.
49. Remillard RL, Modransky PD, Welker FH, et al. Dietary management of cystic calculi in a horse. J Equine Vet Sci 1992;12:359–63.
50. Djurickovic SM, Gandhi D, Brown K, et al. Urolithiasis in baby pigs. Vet Med Small Anim Clin 1973;68:1151–3.
51. Done SH. Urolithiasis in pig units—a gritty problem. Vet J 2004;168:209–10.
52. Halland SK, House JK, George LW. Urethroscopy and laser lithotripsy for the diagnosis and treatment of obstructive urolithiasis in goats and pot-bellied pigs. J Am Vet Med Assoc 2002;220:1831–4.
53. Kakino J, Sato R, Naito Y. Purine metabolism of uric acid urolithiasis induced in newborn piglets. J Vet Med Sci 1998;60:203–20.
54. Maes DGD, Vrielinck J, Nillet S, et al. Urolithiasis in finishing pigs. Vet J 2004;168: 317–22.
55. McIntosh GH. Urolithiasis in animals. Aust Vet J 1978;54:267–71.
56. Capak D, Bedrica L, Vnuk D, et al. Two cases of urolithiasis in rabbits. Tierarztl Umsch 2006;61:20–33.
57. Flatt RE, Carpenter AB. Identification of crystalline material in urine of rabbits. Am J Vet Res 1971;32:655–8.
58. Flemming GJ, Carpenter JW. What is your diagnosis? Large (40x60cm) abdominal mass with a heterogenous mineral opacity. J Am Vet Med Assoc 2000;217:1463–4.
59. McIntosh GH. Urolithiasis in animals. Aust Vet J 1978;54:267–71.
60. Reckler J, Rodman JS, Jacobs D, et al. Urothelial injury to the rabbit bladder from various alkaline and acidic solutions used to dissolve kidney stones. J Urol 1986; 136:181–3.
61. Vannevel J. Formation of urinary calculus in the urethra of a rabbit. Exotic DVM 2002;4:6–7.
62. Jones RJ, Stephenson R, Fountain D, et al. Urolithiasis in a chinchilla. Vet Rec 1995;136:400.
63. Spence S, Skae K. Urolithiasis in a chinchilla. Vet Rec 1995;136:524.
64. Boll RA, Suckow MA, Hawkins EC. Bilateral ureteral calculi in a guinea pig. J Small Exotic Anim Med 1991;1:60–3.
65. Fehr M, Rappold S. Urolithiasis in 20 guinea pigs (Cavia porcellus). Tieraerztliche Praxis 1997;5:543–7.
66. Griffin C. Non-surgical removal of urethral stones in a guinea pig. Exotic DVM 2001;3:13–4.
67. Peng X, Griffith JW, Lang CM. Cystitis, urolithiasis and cystic calculi in ageing guinea pigs. Lab Anim 1990;24:159–63.
68. Stieger S, Wenker C, Ziegler-Gohm D, et al. Ureterolithiasis and papilloma formation in the ureter of a guinea pig. Vet Radiol Ultrasound 2003;44:326–9.
69. Huerkamp MJ, Dillehay DL. Struvite uroliths in a male mouse. Lab Anim Sci 1995; 45:222–4.
70. Wojcinski ZW, Renlund RC, Barsoum NJ, et al. Struvite urolithasis in a B6C3F1 mouse. Lab Anim 1992;26:281–7.

71. Bluestone R, Waisman J, Klinenberg JR. Chronic experimental hyperuricemic nephropathy. Lab Invest 1975;33:273–9.
72. Bushinsky DA, Asplin JR, Grynpas MD, et al. Calcium oxalate stone formation in genetic hypercalciuric stone-forming rats. Kidney Int 2002;61:975–87.
73. Dontas IA, Khaldi L. Urolithiasis and transitional call carcinoma of the bladder in a Wistar rat. J Am Assoc Lab An Sci 2006;45:64–7.
74. Khan SR, Hackett RL. Calcium oxalate urolithiasis in the rats. Is it a model for human stone disease? A review of recent literature. Scan Electron Microsc 1985;2:759–74.
75. Linnemann Kuch P, Schwille PO. Ammonium urate urolithiasis in the rat with portocaval shunt—some aspects of mineral metabolism and urine composition. Urol Res 1986;14:319–22.
76. McIntosh GH. Urolithiasis in animals. Aust Vet J 1978;54:267–71.
77. Mook DM, Painter JA, Pullium JK, et al. Urolithiasis associated with experimental lymphocytic choriomeningitis virus inoculation in lewis rats. Comp Med 2004;54: 318–23.
78. Clark WT, Pass D, Biddle J, et al. Urinary calculi composed of magnesium hydrogen phosphate in a kangaroo. Aust Vet J 1982;59:62–3.
79. Halsey TR. Urethral obstruction due to ammonium urate uroliths in western grey kangaroos. Aust Vet Pract 1996;26:60–4.
80. McFee WE, Osborne CA. Struvite calculus in the vagina of a bottlenose dolphin (*Tursiops truncatus*). J Wildl Dis 2004;40:125–8.
81. Harms CA, Lo Piccolo R, Rotstein DS, et al. Struvite penile urethrolithiasis in a pygmy sperm whale (*Kogia breviceps*). J Wildl Dis 2004;40:588–93.
82. Faltas NH. Urolithiasis in a cynomolgus monkey (*Macaca fascicularis*): a case report. Contemp Top Lab Anim Sci 2000;39:18–9.
83. Lees CJ, Carlson CS, O'Sullivan MG. Urinary calculus caused by plant material in a cynomolgus monkey. Lab Anim Sci 1995;45:441–2.
84. O'Rourke CM, Dw Brammer, Roman GS, et al. Calcium carbonate urolithiasis in an adult male cynomolgus monkey. Lab Anim Sci 1995;45:222–4.
85. Dutton MA. Ammonium acid urate urolith in an iguana. Exotic Pet practice 2000;5:79.
86. McKown RD. A cystic calculus from a wild western spiny softshell turtle (*Apole [trionyx] spiniferus hartwegi*). J Zoo Wildl Med 1998;29:347.
87. Stroud RK. Nephrolithiasis in a harbor seal. J Am Vet Med Assoc 1979;175:924–5.
88. Dennison S, Gulland F, Haulena M, et al. Urate nephrolithiasis in a northern elephant seal (Mirounga angustirostris) and a California sea lion (*Zalophus californianus*). J Zoo Wildl Med 2007;38:114–20.

Changing Paradigms in the Diagnosis of Urolithiasis

Jody P. Lulich, DVM, PhD*, Carl A. Osborne, DVM, PhD

KEYWORDS

- Urolithiasis • Crystalluria • Ultrasonography
- Nephrolithiasis • Proteome

The word "diagnosis" comes from Latin via the Greek word *diagignoskein*, which means to discern or distinguish. Its prefix "dia-" means "through" or "apart." "Gnosis" (*gignoskein*), the root word in diagnosis, means "knowledge." Diagnosis is the process of "clearing, seeing or distinguishing through knowledge." An accurate diagnosis is the foundation for providing appropriate care to mitigate disease. In other words, optimal patient care depends on keen diagnostic acumen and thoughtful analysis of the trade-offs between the benefits and risks of tests and treatments.

"Paradigm" is defined as a model or example. In the context of this article, paradigm is used to refer to a thought pattern (ie, a model of thinking) in the discipline of veterinary medicine. Following this line of reasoning, a "paradigm shift" is a fundamental change from the traditional model of thinking. This article presents four paradigm shifts in the diagnoses of urolithiasis. Because it is the nature of science to continue to refine and explore, the article also provides several paradigm shifts foreshadowing the future.

URINE COLLECTION AND STORAGE FOR RELIABLE CRYSTAL DETECTION
Paradigm

"If the urinalysis cannot be performed within 30 minutes following collection, the sample should be immediately refrigerated to minimize changes caused by bacterial contaminants and autolysis."[1]

Paradigm Shift

"...refrigeration of urine samples enhance in vitro formation of crystals... urine samples stored at refrigeration temperature for 24 hours resulted in the erroneous (false-positive) interpretation in 28% of cats and dogs..."[2]

Veterinary Clinical Sciences Department, Minnesota Urolith Center, College of Veterinary Medicine, University of Minnesota, 1352 Boyd Avenue, St. Paul, MN 55108, USA
* Corresponding author.
E-mail address: lulic001@umn.edu (J.P. Lulich).

Vet Clin Small Anim 39 (2008) 79–91
doi:10.1016/j.cvsm.2008.10.005
0195-5616/08/$ – see front matter © 2008 Elsevier Inc. All rights reserved.

The advent of effective medical protocols to dissolve and prevent uroliths in dogs and cats has resulted in renewed interest in detection and interpretation of crystalluria (**Table 1**). Identification of urine crystals formed in vivo may aid in detection of disorders that predispose animals to urolith formation, estimation of the mineral composition of uroliths when uroliths are not available for analysis, and evaluation of the effectiveness of medical protocols prescribed to dissolve or prevent uroliths. In vivo

Table 1	
Clinical significance of crystalluria	
Significance	**Explanation**
Risk factor for urolith or crystalline-matrix plug formation	Crystal formation indicates that urine is sufficiently saturated such that it could support the formation and growth of uroliths of that respective mineral type. If sufficient numbers of crystals are present, with a concomitant inflammatory process, male cats are at increased risk for matrix-crystalline plug formation. Because crystals have not been demonstrated to cause lower urinary tract signs, crystalluria is an indicator to evaluate the patient for uroliths. However, uroliths can also be present in the absence of urine crystals.
Indication of disease	Crystals also from as a consequence of disease processes altering urine composition. For example, calcium-containing crystals can be present in cats with hypercalcemia. Xanthine crystals may assist the diagnosis of hereditary xanthinuria. Urate crystals may indicate decreased liver function.
Predict mineral composition of uroliths/plugs	Crystals in the urine of cats and dogs are often similar to the minerals identified in uroliths and urethral plugs of the corresponding patient. However, crystal identification is not an accurate substitute for quantitative mineral analysis.
Index of therapeutic response	Formation of crystals and uroliths are dependent on production of urine that is oversaturated for that particular mineral. One strategy to reduce urolith recurrence is to enhance the solubility of that mineral salt in urine. The presence of crystals consistent with the composition of previous uroliths, indicates that urine saturation has not been sufficiently reduced.

To minimize in vitro or iatrogenic crystal formation, urine should be analyzed before administration of therapy (except when evaluating therapeutic response), analyzed within 1 to 2 hours of collection from the urinary bladder, and stored at room temperature in a container such that the surface of the urine sample is not exposed to air (eg, stored in a capped syringe).

factors that predispose cats and dogs to crystalluria include the concentration and water solubility of crystallogenic substances in urine, urine pH, and the rate of urine flow.

Unfortunately, in vitro changes in urine composition that develop after sample collection may promote formation of the same types of crystals that form in vivo. Thus, caution must be used in clinical interpretation of crystals found in urine sediment, as these may not have been present when the sample was collected. In vitro factors that may influence formation of crystals in urine specimens include temperature, time, evaporation, urine pH, and growth of microbial contaminants that produce urease.

Examination of urine samples within a short time after collection minimizes in vitro crystal formation and other undesirable in vitro effects that interfere with accurate interpretation of routine urinalyses. The objective is to anaylze urine samples with in vitro laboratory characteristics that closely resemble in vivo characteristics of urine. In the event that diagnostic evaluation of urine after specimen collection is delayed, refrigeration of samples is commonly recommended.[1] Refrigeration preserves many of the physical and chemical properties of urine, as well as morphologic characteristics of urine sediment. It also minimizes in vitro growth of microbes. However, clinical observations suggest that refrigeration enhances in vitro crystal formation. In one study, urine specimens were collected from 8 cats and 31 dogs.[2] In vitro formation of calcium oxalate crystals was observed in urine samples from one cat and eight dogs. When urine was stored at room temperature, in vitro calcium oxalate crystal formation was detected in one of nine aliquots at 6 hours, and two of nine aliquots at 24 hours. In urine samples that were stored at refrigeration temperature, in vitro calcium oxalate crystal formation was detected in four of nine aliquots at 6 hours, and in all nine aliquots at 24 hours. In two dogs, in vitro formation of magnesium ammonium phosphate crystals was observed in aliquots of urine stored for 6 and 24 hours at room and refrigeration temperatures. In vitro crystals formed less frequently in urine samples stored at room temperature.

In another study of 10 healthy beagle dogs, only in vitro struvite crystals were observed following refrigeration for 24 hours.[3] Similarly, in vitro formation of only struvite crystals was reported in a study to evaluate the effect of refrigeration on urine samples from cats.[4] Refrigeration may promote in vitro csytalluria because temperature-dependent electrostatic attractions between water molecules and calculogenic ions play an important role in crystal formation. As temperature decreases, water molecules are less likely to flow and disrupt the attraction between ions that are capable of forming crystals. To minimize in vitro artifacts when delay of analysis of urine samples is anticipated, collect a volume of urine sufficient to provide aliquots for storage at both refrigeration and room temperatures. This maneuver should minimize false-positive crystalluria, yet still preserve the remaining microscopic features of the sediment.

EFFECTIVE MEDICAL IMAGING
Paradigm

" …we believe that cystosonography may replace radiography in detecting cystic calculi in the majority of patients."[5]

Paradigm Shift

"Although ultrasonography is gaining in popularity as a sensitive and safe method to detect uroliths, the information obtained should be considered complimentary to survey radiology and not a potential diagnostic replacement stated Drs. Lulich and Osborne."

In 1993, Dr Karoly Voros and colleagues made the following statement about diagnostic ultrasonography, "...we believe that cystosonography may replace radiography in detecting cystic calculi in the majority of patients."[5] Almost two decades later, their prediction is not far from reality. Ultrasonography is gaining popularity as a sophisticated diagnostic tool. Results of an in vitro study concluded that ultrasonography was more sensitive than survey and contrast cystography for detection of urocystoliths (**Table 2**).[6] Furthermore, the operator and patient are not exposed to ionizing radiation. Over the past two decades, the quality of the image has continued to improve and the price of ownership has continued to decline. These factors position utlrasonography as a cost-effective tool for the general practitioner. However, if ultrasound becomes the sole method of urolith detection, several important diagnostic features of uroliths would be overlooked, most importantly the information to accurately predict mineral composition.[7]

Accurately predicting the mineral composition of uroliths before their removal and analysis will permit veterinarians to develop rational therapeutic plans with reliable outcomes. Consider the following example of a 2-year-old male Havanese and Bichon mixed-breed dog. Because this patient had hematuria and pollakiuria, abdominal ultrasonography was performed. A 1.3-mm urolith was detected in the urinary bladder (**Fig. 1**). Is ultrasonographic information sufficient to recommend therapy? Should the urolith be removed surgically? Before surgery, a survey abdominal radiograph was performed; a faintly radio-opaque, smooth, round urocystolith was identified. Additional uroliths were not detected in the urethra (see **Fig. 1**). What is the best prediction of the composition of the urolith? Should serum concentrations of bile acids be evaluated before surgical urolith removal? If surgical urolith removal will be performed

Table 2
False-negative urolith-detection rates of medical imaging procedures for identifying urocystoliths in an in vitro model

Detection Method	Urolith Type						
	CaP (n = 40)	CaOx (n = 118)	Cystine (n = 148)	MAP (n = 60)	Silica (n = 59)	Urate (n = 108)	All (n = 179)
Survey radiography	25%	5%	27%	2%	5%	22%	13%
Pneumocystography	5%	5%	2%	0%	8%	13%	6%
Double-contrast cystography[a]	8%	7%	0%	0%	0%	7%	4%
Ultrasonography[b]	2%	2%	6%	0%	2%	7%	3%

Urolith size was not standard for each mineral type, but represented submissions to the Minnesota Urolith Center in 1991 of uroliths retrieved from dogs with spontaneous disease. Evaluators were masked to the contents of the phantom bladder for all detection methods except ultrasonography; consequently, operator bias may contribute to lower false-negative detection rates associated with ultrasonography.

Abbreviations: CaOx, calcium oxalate; CaP, calcium phosphate; MAP = magnesium ammonium phosphate.

[a] Approximate concentration of positive contrast agent = 200 mg/mL; lower concentrations (ie, 80 mg/mL) were associated with greater false negatives.

[b] Evaluation obtained using a 7.5 MHz transducer; lower frequency transducers (ie, 5.0 MHz and 3.5 MHz) were associated with greater false negatives.

Data from Weichselbaum RC, Feeney DA, Jessen CR, et al. Urocystolith detection: comparison of survey, contrast radiographic and ultrasonographic techniques in an in vitro bladder phantom. Vet Radiol Ultrasound 1999;40:386–400.

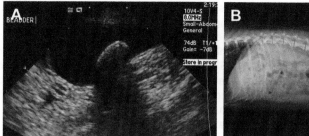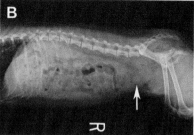

Fig. 1. Ultrasonography of the urinary bladder of a 2-year-old mixed breed dog revealed a 1.3-cm intraluminal object with distal shadowing (A). These findings are consistent with a urocystolith. Survey radiograph of the same patient determined that the stone was minimally radio-opaque (B).

following administration of anesthetic agents that require hepatic elimination, if the severity of liver failure is of sufficient magnitude such that hemostasis is impaired, or if nonsteroidal anti-inflammatory drugs will be prescribed to manage postsurgical pain, the answer should be yes. To avoid the complications of anesthetizing a patient with probable liver failure, this information is essential to plan for a successful outcome. Presurgical serum concentrations of bile acids were obtained. The patient's fasting value was 47 umol/L (normal is less than 6) and the postprandial was 119 umol/L (normal is less than 15). Abdominal ultrasonography was repeated looking for a vascular shunt, but one was not detected. During surgery a mesenteric portogram was performed; multiple extrahepatic vascular shunts were revealed. An accurate prediction of the composition of this urolith and thoughtful planning resulted in a successful outcome. The urolith was submitted for analysis; it was composed of 100% ammonium acid urate (**Fig. 2**).

When predicting mineral composition of uroliths many factors are used. Some veterinarians primarily rely on identification of crystal type. However, crystalluria is not a consistent feature of the urinalysis in dogs and cats with uroliths. For example, in one study of 30 cases of struvite urocystoliths in cats, struvite crystals were only detected in 17 patients.[8]

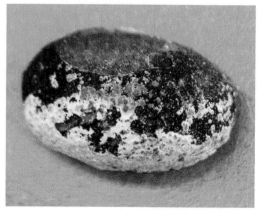

Fig. 2. Urosyctolith removed from the dog depicted in Fig. 1. The stone was composed of 100% ammonium acid urate.

Predicting mineral composition from survey radiographs offers many advantages because multiple pieces of information (eg, radio-opacity, uniformity of radio-opacity, shape, and surface contour) are processed from a single test (**Tables 3** and **4**). In addition to mineral composition, urolith number, size, and location can aid to selection of therapy. For example, uroliths less than 5 mm in diameter are easily removed by voiding urohydropropulsion or basket retrieval in most dogs. Urethroliths, however, which are usually missed or not evaluated during routine ultrasound, cannot be managed by voiding urohydropropulsion of stone basket retrieval. Although ultrasonography is gaining in popularity as a sensitive and safe method to detect uroliths, the information obtained should be considered complimentary to survey radiology instead of a replacement (**Table 5**).

RELIABLE DETECTION OF INCOMPLETE UROLITH REMOVAL
Paradigm

"Palpation of the bladder neck and passage of a catheter through the urethra are indicated to ensure that the bladder neck or urethra is not blocked by calculi. Repeat flushing and aspiration are indicated to remove all discrete calculi and small particles of sand."[9]

Paradigm Shift

"Omission of radiographs (to verify that all uroliths were removed following cystotomy) falls below the standard of care."[10]

Recurrence of uroliths following surgery is commonly attributed to failure of medical therapy to adequately reduce factors promoting urolith formation. However, this hypothesis is based on the premise that all stones were completely removed from the urinary tract before therapeutic intervention. Consider the following observations. The authors performed a retrospective study evaluating the efficacy of cystotomies to remove urocystoliths from 37 dogs and 29 cats in the authors' veterinary teaching hospital.[11] Incomplete removal of uroliths was documented in eight dogs and four cats. The observation that uroliths were detected in the lower urinary tract immediately following cystotomy in 20% of cats and 14% of dogs in a teaching hospital with board certified surgeons on the staff emphasizes an inherent risk associated with this procedure. Based on consultations with the authors' colleagues in private practice, incomplete removal of uroliths occurred more frequently than has been recognized. A common theme is discovery of the remaining uroliths several weeks or months following surgery, when patients are re-evaluated because of persistent or recurrent signs of lower urinary tract disease. In this situation, delayed detection of uroliths is often erroneously attributed to recurrence (pseudorecurrence). This in turn may result in inaccurate and inappropriate prognostic and therapeutic recommendations to prevent future recurrence because the most common cause for rapid recurrence of uroliths—that is, incomplete surgical removal—was often overlooked.

Although commonly recognized following surgical removal of uroliths, pseudorecurrence can also occur when uroliths are eradicated by other modalities (eg, medical dissolution, voiding urohydropropulsion, laproscopic-assisted cystotomy, lithotripsy, and so forth). Avoiding incomplete urolith removal requires a high degree of suspicion because even with the best surgical techniques, some uroliths commonly evade detection and removal. To minimize this complication, the following should be considered:

Normograde and retrograde passage of urinary catheters is a common method of assessing complete urolith removal. However, it is the authors' opinion that retrograde transurethral catheterization is insensitive when used in this manner. This is especially

Table 3
Predicting mineral composition of canine uroliths based on radiographic appearance

Mineral	Radiographic Opacity Compared with Soft Tissue	Surface Contour	Shape	Usual Number	Approximate Size
CaOx monohydrate	+++ to ++++	Smooth	Commonly round	>20	2 mm–7mm
CaOx dihydrate	+++ to ++++	Rough	Rosette	>5, few large single	1 mm–15 mm
Sterile MAP	++ to +++	Irregular, few smooth	Round to ovoid	1–3	5 mm–15 mm
Infection MAP	+ to +++	Smooth to slightly rough	Round to faceted or pryamidal	>4 to many	4 mm to >20 mm
Urate	– to ++	Smooth	Round to oval	Few or too numerous to count	1 mm–15 mm
CaP	+++ to ++++	Smooth	Round to cuboidal	Many, some few	2 mm–6 mm
Cystine	– to +++	Smooth to bosselated	Round	Many to few	2 mm–10 mm
Silica	++ to ++++	Smooth	Radiating spokes	One or many	2 mm–10 mm
Xanthine	– to +	Smooth	Round to ovoid	Few to many	1 mm–4 mm

Abbreviations: CaOx = calcium oxalate; CaP=calcium phosphate; MAP = magnesium ammonium phosphate.

Table 4
Predicting mineral composition of feline uroliths based on radiographic appearance

Mineral	Radiographic Opacity Compared with Soft Tissue	Surface Contour	Shape	Usual Number	Approximate Size
CaOx monohydrate	+++ to ++++	Smooth, but occasionally bosselated	Commonly round, but also rosette	>5	1 mm–5 mm
CaOx dihydrate	+++ to ++++	Rough to smooth	Rosettes	>3	1 mm–7 mm
Sterile MAP	++ to +++	Slightly rough	Round or discoid	Usually 1–3, occassionally many	3 mm–10 mm
Infection MAP	+ to +++	Smooth to slightly rough	Round to faceted	Few to many	2 to >7 mm
Urate	– to ++	Smooth	Round to ovoid	Usually 1, but up to 5	2 mm–10 mm
CaP	+++ to ++++	Rough	To rare to comment	Too rare to comment	1 mm–4 mm
Cystine	– to +++	Rough	Round	Many, but some with few	1 mm–4 mm
Silica	++ to ++++	To rare to comment	To rare to comment	Too rare to comment	1 mm–4 mm
Xanthine	– to +	Smooth	Round to ovoid	1–3	1 mm–5mm

Table 5
Comparing the ability survey radiography and ultrasonography to detect urolith features

Urolith Feature	Survey Radiography	Ultrasonography
Radio-opacity	++++	−
Variations in radio-opacity	+++	−
Shape	+++	+
Surface contour	+++	−
Diameter	+++	+++
Number	+ to +++	+ to ++
Location		
Kidney	+++	+++
Ureter	+++	+
Bladder	+++	++++
Urethra	+++	+

true for uroliths with an irregular contour (eg, calcium oxalate and silica) that allow catheters and flushing solutions to slide past when lodged in the urethral lumen.

Radiography is a valuable technique in the diagnosis of incomplete urolith removal. In fact, it is the standard of care. In a recent case review by PLIT, the Professional Liability Insurance Trust for the American Veterinary Medical Association, a veterinarian who does not perform radiography to verify complete removal of uroliths following cystotomy is practicing substandard care.[10] Therefore, the authors recommend that appropriate medical imaging be performed following cystotomy to verify complete urolith removal.[12]

The ability to detect uroliths following surgery by radiography depends on their size, location, and mineral composition. Although survey radiography is suitable for identification of radio-opaque uroliths greater than approximately 2 mm to 3 mm in diameter, contrast-enhanced procedures are needed to identify uroliths composed of compounds similar to the radiographic density of soft tissue (eg, ammonium urate, cystine, xanthine). For these cases, double-contrast cystography is the preferred technique because it has been associated with high sensitivity and low false negative-detection rates. Although a caveat commonly cited in the context that use of room air is the cause of formation of air emboli, the risk of this complication has been uncommon in the authors' clinical experience. In patients with substantial hemorrhage from the lower urinary tract, informed consent and use of carbon dioxide (CO_2 refills and dispenser, Genuine Innovations, Tuczon AZ) or nitrous oxide may be considered to minimize the risk of air embolization. Following instillation of negative contrast agent, the authors inject 1 mL to 6 mLs of iodinated contrast material, depending on bladder size. One report suggested a minimum of three orthogonal views to evaluate the urinary bladder: left and right lateral and a ventrodorsal view. In the authors' experience, the most cost-effective postoperative technique to evaluate the urinary bladder is use of two lateral views, one before and one following instillation of negative and positive contrast agents. In some cases, stones lodged in the pelvic urethral obviate radiographic detection because they become obscured by the bones of the pelvis. If this is likely, rectal palpation of the pelvic urethra should be sufficient to detect their presence. The authors rarely suggest ultrasound as a means of evaluation immediately following surgery because additional air in the abdomen and location of stones in the urethra limit its usefulness to accurately evaluate the entire urinary tract.

RECOGNIZING ADDITONAL CAUSES FOR KIDNEY DISEASE
Paradigm

"In only a small percentage of all cases of urinary stone disease in dogs and cats are calculi located in the renal pelvis."[13]

Paradigm Shift

"A 10-fold increase in the frequency of upper tract uroliths occurred in cats during the 20-year interval (1980 to 1990)."[14]

Until the 1990s, the prevailing opinion was that uroliths uncommonly affected the upper urinary tract of dogs and cats. Furthermore, the occurrence of calcium oxalate nephroliths was considered to be rare. However, results of a study performed at the Minnesota Urolith Center revealed a 10-fold increase in the frequency of upper tract uroliths in cats evaluated at nine veterinary teaching hospitals in the United States during the 20-year study period.

The increased prevalence in upper urinary tract uroliths has created new diagnostic considerations and challenges. For example, in a study of 88 cats with chronic kidney disease, 41 (47%) had upper-tract stones.[15,16] Of these 41 cats, 10% had ureteroliths. These findings indicate the need to perform medical imaging in cats, and potentially dogs, with chronic kidney disease.

When developing a diagnostic plan to determine whether or not a urolith is obstructing a ureter, several factors, including the sensitivity of the diagnostic procedure, the status of the patient's renal function, and the type of therapy (medical or surgical) need to be considered. Although survey abdominal radiographs are of value in providing an overview of the entire urinary tract and surrounding abdominal structures, they cannot be relied upon to verify partial or total obstruction of ureters with uroliths.

Intravenous urography is a sensitive method to detect ureteral obstruction in nonazotemic and mildly azotemic patients. Excretion of radio-opaque contrast agent by the kidneys is dependent on adequate glomerular filtration. In patients with marked azotemia, reduced filtration of contrast media may impair visualization of the kidneys, ureters, and bladder. This can be overcome by increasing the dose of contrast media administered[15] and increasing the time of the procedure (ie, additional radiographs obtained 2 to 4 hours after administration of contrast media). To minimize adverse events associated with intravenously administered contrast media, the authors recommend that deficits in hydration be corrected before their administration. Adverse reactions to contrast media can also be minimized by use of nonionic iodinated contrast media (eg, iothalamate meglumine).

To minimize the risk of contrast media-induced nephropathy, consider transcutaneous antegrade contrast pyelography as an alternative to intravenous urography.[17] Contrast-enhanced pyelography provides a sensitive method of verifying the presence and location of ureteral obstruction. However, puncturing the renal pelvis to inject contrast media may reduce intraureteral pressure. Increased hydrostatic pressure proximal to the site of obstruction may promote movement of the urolith through the lumen of the ureter.[18] Therefore, in some patients it may be advantageous to delay transcutaneous antegrade contrast-enhanced pyelography until noninvasive strategies to promote movement of stones through the ureter have been evaluated. However, in situations where intravenous urography is likely to be unsatisfactory because of severe renal dysfunction (ie, the patient is severely azotemic), transcutaneous antegrade pyelography should be considered. Sedation is required to perform contrast pyelography. As an alternative to evaluating severely azotemic patients by contrast radiography, the authors recommend a combination of survey radiography and ultrasonography. Ultrasound findings associated with obstruction of a ureter include a dilation of the renal pelvis, dilation of the ureter, and a high-resistive index.

PARADIGM SHIFTS FORESHADOWING THE FUTURE
Genetic Tests to Identify Risk Factors for Urolith Formation

Persistent crystalluria, a marker of urine supersatruation, has been commonly used to identify patients at increased risk for urolithiasis. However, the reliability of this marker to discriminate between stone-formers and those unlikely to from stones is debatable. This is because urine supersaturation for some crystal types occurs in clinically healthy dogs and cats. However, the availability of the canine genome and the availability of the feline genome in the near future will provide opportunities for a paradigm shift in the possibilities to identify urolith-formers now and in the future. DNA testing is currently available to indentify Newfoundland and Labrador dogs at risk for cystine urolithiasis (see the article by Bannasch and Henthorn elsewhere in this issue.) Expect similar diagnostic advancements for dogs and cats with other urolith types.

Proteomic Biomarker Discovery

Urine represents a rich source of information related to the functioning of many processes, including those associated with urolithiasis. Analyzing the protein/peptide composition of urine and uroliths can provide information as to the peptide structures actively participating in the construction of, the building blocks for, and "innocent bystander" proteins incorporated into the matrix of urinary stones.

Proteomics represents the simultaneous characterization of a large number of proteins in tissue, cells, or fluid, and in the authors' case, urine. The proteome is the protein/peptide compliment of all actively expressed genes with the addition of those generated through their posttranslational modification (ie, phosphorylation, ubiquitination, methylation, acetylation, glycosylation, oxidation, nitrosylation, and so forth). In some instances, protein products of historically expressed genes may also be present. However, this is less likely, as urine is regularly voided.

The relevance of this diagnostic approach rests on several tenets: (1) each gene is translated into one or several protein isoforms; (2) the protein makeup of urine closely reflects the activity of the fluid and the processes governing urolith formation; and (3) each pathologic process results from abnormal synthesis, impaired degradation, or mishandling of proteins participating in the functional makeup of urine. Therefore, detection of a specific protein/peptide ensemble should provide a signature of a particular pathologic process. Moreover, such signatures may be detected before any clinical manifestation of disease.

The core technology permitting urinary proteomic analysis is the mass spectrometer. This technological platform permits detection of multiple proteins/peptides in unprocessed or minimally processed urine in minutes. In one study, surface-enhanced laser desorption/ionization time-of-flight mass spectroscopic analysis of urine and uroliths from dogs resulted in unique peptide profiles discriminating struvite, calcium oxalate, and urate stone formers.[19] To further advance this systems approach of discovery, metabolic profiling through proton nuclear magnetic spectroscopic analysis is available to provide information on the metabolic processes responsible for the changes in urine.[20,21] These more comprehensive analyses are redefining what we call "normal" urine.

REFERENCES

1. Osborne CA, Stevens JB. Urine Sediment: under the microscope. In: Osborne CA, Stevens JB, editors. Urinalysis: guide to compassionate patient care. Shawnee Mission (KS): Bayer Co; 1999. p. 125–50.
2. Albasan H, Lulich JP, Osborne CA, et al. Effects of storage time and temperature on pH, specific gravity, and crystal formation in urine samples from dogs and cats. J Am Vet Med Assoc 2003;222:176–9.
3. Duderstadt JM, Weingand KW. Effects of overnight refrigeration on routine dog urinalysis. Proceedings of the 25th Annual Meeting American Society for Veterinary Clinical Pathology. Orlando, FL, November 14–17, 1990.
4. Sturgess CP, Hesford A, Owen H, et al. An investigation into the effects of storage on the diagnosis of crystalluria in cats. J Feline Med Surg 2001;3:81–5.
5. K Voros, Wladar S, Vrabely T, et al. Ultrasonographic diagnosis of urinary bladder calculi in dogs. Canine Practice 1993;18:29–33.
6. Weichselbaum RC, Feeney DA, Jessen CR, et al. Urocystolith detection: comparison of survey, contrast radiographic and ultrasonographic techniques in an in vitro bladder phantom. Vet Radiol Ultrasound 1999;40:386–400.
7. Weichselbaum RC, Feeney DA, Jessen CR, et al. Loss of urocystolith architectural clarity during in vivo radiographic simulation versus in vitro visualization. Vet Radiol Ultrasound 2000;41:241–6.
8. Osborne CA, Lulich JP, Kruger JM, et al. Medical dissolution of feline struvite urocystoliths. J Am Vet Med Assoc 1990;196:1053–63.
9. Waldron DR. Urinary bladder. In: Slatter D, editor. Textbook of Small Animal Surgery. 2nd edition. Philadelphia: W. B. Saunders Co; 1993. p. 1458.
10. Omission of radiograph falls below standard of care. A Report for PLIT-Sponsored for Professional Liability Program Participants. Summer 2005;24(3):1–3.
11. Lulich JP, Perrine L, Osborne CA, et al. Postsurgical recurrence of calcium oxalate uroliths in dogs. J Vet Intern Med 1992;6:119.
12. Lulich JP, Osborne CA. Incomplete urolith removal: prevention, detection, and correction. In: Bonagura JD, Twedt DC, editors. Kirk's current veterinary therapy XIV, Small animal practice. Philadelphia: W.B Saunders Co; 2009. p. 936–9.
13. Ling GV. Nephrolithiasis: prevalence of mineral type. In: Bonagura JD, editor. Kirk's current veterinary therapy XII, Small animal practice. Philadelphia: W. B Saunders Co; 1995. p. 980.
14. Lekcharoensuk C, Osborne CA, Lulich JP, et al. Evaluation of trends in the frequency of calcium oxalate uroliths in the upper urinary tract of cats. J Am Anim Hosp Assoc 2005;41:39–46.
15. Polzin DJ, Ross SJ, Osborne CA, et al. Urolithiasis and feline renal failure part II, in Proceedings. 21st Annual American College of Veterinary Internal Medicine Forum 2003;785–6.
16. Johnston GR, Walter PA, Feeney DA. Diagnostic imaging of the urinary tract. In: Osborne CA,, Finco DR, editors. Canine and feline nephrology and urology. Baltimore (MD): Williams and Wilkins; 1995. p. 230–76.
17. Adin CA, Herrgesell EJ, Nyland TG, et al. Antegrade pyelography for suspected ureteral obstruction in cats: 11 cases 1995–2001. Journal of the American Veterinary Medical Association 2003;222:1576–81.
18. Sivula A, Lehtonen T. Spontaneous passage of artificial concretions applied in the rabbit ureter. Scand J urol Nephrol 1967;1:259–63.
19. Forterre S, Raila J, Kohn B, et al. Protein profiling of organic stone matrix and urine from dogs with urolithiasis. J Anim Physiol Nutr 2006;90:192–9.

20. Beckonert O, Keun HC, Ebbels TMD, et al. Metabolic profiling, metabolomic and metabonomic procedures for NMR spectroscopy of urine, plasma, serum and tissue extracts. Nat Protoc 2007;2:2692–703.
21. Wevers RA, Engelke UFH, Moolenaar SH, et al. H-NMR spectroscopy of body fluids: inborn errors of purine and pyrimidine metabolism. Clin Chem 1999;45: 539–48.

Changing Paradigms in Ethical Issues and Urolithiasis

Carl A. Osborne, DVM, PhD[a],*, Jody P. Lulich, DVM, PhD[a],
James F. Wilson, DVM, JD[b], Carroll H. Weiss[c]

KEYWORDS

• Ethics • Pseudorecurrence • Uroliths • Calculi • Golden rule
• Quantitative urolith analysis • Malpractice

DEFINITIONS OF TERMS AND CONCEPTS

Profession

How would you define the term "profession"? How does it differ from other occupations? A profession has been defined as an occupation that: (1) regulates itself through systematic required education or collegial discipline; (2) has a base in technical, specialized knowledge, and (3) has a service, rather than a profit orientation, enshrined in an ethical code.[1]

Ethics

How would you define the term "ethic"? The word ethic is derived from the Greek word *ethos*, meaning character or custom. It implies conforming to moral standards or conforming to the standards of conduct of a given profession. To be ethical, one must be in accord with some moral standard or code of conduct. The term "moral" is derived from the Latin word *moralis*, which signifies manners. Morality deals with or makes a distinction between right or wrong conduct. It implies conforming to a standard of right behavior. Synonyms for moral include the terms "virtue" and "ethic." Law is not a synonym for morality.

Veterinary Medical Ethics

The original United States Veterinary Medical Association Code of Ethics was adopted in 1867.[2] Now, broad-based and general principles of veterinary medical ethics have been adopted by the American Veterinary Medical Association (AVMA).[2] They

[a] Veterinary Clinical Sciences Department, Minnesota Urolith Center, College of Veterinary Medicine, University of Minnesota, 1352 Boyd Avenue, St. Paul, MN 55108, USA
[b] Priority Veterinary Management Consultants, 116 South Main Street, Yardley, PA 19067, USA
[c] DCA Study Group on Urinary Stones, Dalmatian Club of America, 8290 Northwest 26th Place, Sunrise, FL, USA
* Corresponding author.
E-mail address: osbor002@umn.edu (C.A. Osborne).

Vet Clin Small Anim 39 (2008) 93–109
doi:10.1016/j.cvsm.2008.10.007
0195-5616/08/$ – see front matter © 2008 Elsevier Inc. All rights reserved.

vetsmall.theclinics.com

encompass such topics as guidelines for professional behavior, advertising, fees, referrals, consultations, relationship with clients, and various other aspects of the practice of veterinary medicine.[3] Ethical principles governing the practice of veterinary medicine are often more stringent than legal controls. However, they do not cover all facets of veterinary medicine. The ultimate test of our ethics as veterinarians is the conduct that ethical principles dictate or inspire. The ultimate challenge of our behavior is to choose the best course of conduct or action when existing laws or government rules and guidelines do not apply.

The AVMA made the following statement about the "Principles of Veterinary Medical Ethics" (note the emphasis on the Golden Rule): "Exemplary professional conduct upholds the dignity of the veterinary profession. All veterinarians are expected to adhere to a progressive code of ethical conduct known as the Principles of Veterinary Medical Ethics. The basis of the Principles is the Golden Rule. Veterinarians should accept this rule as a guide to their general conduct and abide by the Principles. They should conduct their professional and personal affairs in an ethical manner."[2]

The Golden Rule and Ethics

Can you recite the Golden Rule from memory? Recall that the Golden Rule is a rule of ethical conduct from Matthew 7:12 and Luke 6:31, stating that we should do for others as we would have others do for us. A version of this principle is attributed to the Chinese philosopher Confucius (551–479 BC), who said, "What you do not want done to yourself, do not do to others."[4] Compared with the Biblical version, this version is negative (do not do to others) rather than positive (do to others).

Practicing the positive version of the Golden Rule means that we must take the initiative in being altruistic (having unselfish concern for the welfare of others). Altruism (the opposite of egoism) demands that we consider the interest of others when we use our talents and possessions. Thus, the Golden Rule is of little value unless we recognize that the first move is ours. To practice the Golden Rule, we must strive to put ourselves in others' shoes, paws, hooves, or claws.[5]

When we offer to provide the type of care for our patients that we would select for ourselves, then at the very least our clients know that our primary motive for doing so is based on the Golden Rule. Clients are more likely to have confidence in our recommendations and comply with them if they know that our actions are based on serving their best interests.

Ethical Prognosis and Evidence-Based Medicine

Dorland's Medical Dictionary defines prognosis as "a forecast of the probable outcome of an attack of disease" or "the prospect as to recovery from a disease as indicated by the nature and symptoms of the case."[6] Synonyms for the term prognosis include prediction, foretelling, and forecast.

In context of prognoses, effective communication between clients and doctors cannot consistently occur unless there is mutual understanding. Therefore, in place of poorly defined prognostic terms that are highly subjective, the authors recommend terminology that leads to quantification of the probability of a predicted outcome (**Table 1**). The goal is to help our clients fully understand the message we are trying to convey to them.

Prognosis of diseases requires judgment in the absence of certainty. Therefore, when formulating prognoses, we must remember that "almost right" is still wrong. For some patients, prognoses are life saving; for others they are a death sentence. Therefore, our decisions about the care of our patients should be based on the same conscientious, explicit, and judicious use of current best evidence (so-called "evidence-based medicine") that we would desire physicians to use in caring for us

Table 1 Definition of prognostic terms		
	Prediction of Recovery	
Term	Qualitative	Quantitative %
Excellent	Highly probable	75–100
Good	Probable	50–75
Guarded	Unpredictable	50
Poor	Improbable	25–50
Grave	Highly improbable	0–25

if we were in a similar situation. Putting evidence-based medicine into practice means integrating our individual clinical expertise with the best available external clinical evidence derived from systematic research. The following Grades are recommended to score the strength and the quality of available external evidence:

Grade I evidence is defined as the highest quality evidence. It is derived from at least one properly randomized controlled clinical study.
Grade II evidence may be data obtained from:
At least one well-designed clinical study without randomization;
Cohort or case-controlled analytic studies;
Studies using acceptable laboratory models or simulations in the target species, preferably from more than one center;
Multiple time series; or
Dramatic results in uncontrolled studies.
Grade III evidence is defined as the weakest form of evidence, and may be derived from:
Opinions from respected authorities on the basis of clinical experience;
Descriptive studies;
Studies in other species;
Pathophysiological justification; or
Reports of expert committees.[7,8]

Medical diagnoses are often a matter of educated opinion rather than a matter of fact. It is one thing to make a diagnosis and another thing to substantiate it. Absence of clinical evidence of suspected diseases is not always synonymous with evidence of absence of these diseases. Likewise, detection of evidence that is consistent with a specific type of disease is not always pathognomonic for that specific disease. It follows that we as veterinarians should convey to our clients that our prognoses (and diagnoses) are based on probability, and therefore are not infallible.

Veterinary Medical Ethics and Hippocrates

Hippocrates provided the following advice to his colleagues: "As to diseases, make a habit of two things—to help, or at least do no harm."[9] When confronted with situations in which therapeutic options are associated with significant risk to the patient, we must use caution to avoid the mindset of "Just don't stand there—do something." Why? Because, although the psychologic pressure imposed on veterinarians to do something is occasionally overwhelming, our desire to do something must be evaluated in light of the potential benefits and risks to the patient. There are times when it is in the patient's best interest to "Don't just do something—stand there."[10] We must not misplace emphasis on what treatment to prescribe when the fundamental question is whether or not to prescribe.

Medical Ethics and Professional Competency

We should strive for a realistic view of our professional competency and technical skill. When uncertainty exists as to whether a particular drug or medical or surgical procedure is in the best interests of our patients, we should contemplate the answers to the following questions:

> Based on available information and my knowledge of my own skill and experience with this type of problem, would I consent to the proposed therapeutic plan of action if I were in this patient's situation?
> What therapeutic goals are likely to be achieved?
> If I follow the proposed plan of action, in all probability will the overall benefits justify the associated risks and costs?

Ethics and Referrals

Treating our patients as we would be treated also encompasses patient referrals. No veterinarian has perfect knowledge, understanding, and wisdom about all health care problems. Will Rogers' statement applies: "We are all ignorant, only on different subjects."[4] It is unethical to mislead a client by indicating ability to manage a case, which is beyond our expertise or the capability of our veterinary practice. Clients must be clearly advised about benefit and risk probabilities in such situations. When specialty care or overnight emergency care is reasonably available, ethics requires that the alternatives of these options be discussed with the clients. We must also strive to be aware of the client's ability to pay for veterinary services. Rather than recommending continued long-term care that is of questionable efficacy, it may be more ethical to refer patients to appropriate specialists with the goal of rapid diagnostic resolution and more effective case management. In addition to improved patient care, overall costs may be lower.

Timely discussion of the option of referral is especially relevant when the needs of the patient clearly exceed the expertise of the veterinarian, specialty or overnight care is reasonably available, and clients have expressed the desire for the best possible care. If primary care practitioners know, or should know, that a patient's illness is beyond their knowledge or technical expertise to treat with a reasonable likelihood of success, they are ethically obligated to offer their clients the timely option of consulting specialists or professionals qualified in advanced methods of treatment. Failure to advise his or her client of this option in a timely fashion could lead to allegations of professional negligence (also known as malpractice).

Three common complaints made by clients about referrals are, 1) failure of veterinarians to mention the availability of specialty or overnight emergency veterinary care, 2) procrastination until the patient's problems have become too advanced to be helped by a referral, and 3) the pronouncement "I'm sorry but your pet died overnight" when clients learn after the fact that supervision at an emergency facility was within easy driving distance. When the course of diagnosis or therapy of a patient is not clear, and when the client expresses the desire for the best possible patient care, a referral or consultation must be legally and ethically offered as an option.

Ethics and Profits

If we apply the Golden Rule, we should be on guard to maintain our ethical balance so as not to tip the scales toward caring more about our personal income or profits than about our patients. We must use caution not to lose our balance to the extent that fee advancement becomes detrimental to the management of our patients. To this end, our actions should demonstrate that the humane aspects of veterinary medicine are just as important, if not more so, than financial considerations.

We are all members of a profession whose mission is to foster the well being of others. Our mission is to serve, not to be served. Therefore the true importance of what we do should be measured in the context of what it accomplishes in behalf of others, not just in light of what it does for us in terms of prestige or personal and professional gain.

Practicality and Ethics

To put knowledge and wisdom into practice emphasizes the importance of practicality. However, our commitment to practicality should not be misdirected. Practicality may be a virtue, provided we do not hide behind it as an excuse for ignorance.

Can you recite the Golden Rule? It is probable that most of us have committed the Golden Rule to memory. This being the case, the next question for us to contemplate daily is, "Do our actions reveal that we are committed to putting the Golden Rule into practice?"

Iatrogenic

The Greek term *iatros* means "physician" and is derived from the word *iasthai*, which means to heal or cure. In modern usage " -iatric," and " iatro- " connote a relationship to medical or surgical treatments. What is the meaning of the word "iatrogenic"? The term iatrogenic contains the root word "iatros" and the root word "gennan," which means "to create or produce." *Dorland's Medical Dictionary* defines iatrogenic as any adverse condition or complication in a patient occurring as a result of treatment by a physician.[11] Because there is no comparable English word for adverse events in patients resulting from treatment by veterinarians, the word iatrogenic has been adopted by our profession. The fact that iatrogenic is considered as a pathophysiologic mechanism of disease emphasizes that there are some patients we cannot help, but there are none we cannot harm.

TREATING UROLITHS
Illustrative Case Report

A 4-year-old neutered male Dalmatian (Jake), with a history of ammonium urate urolithiasis, was admitted to a veterinary hospital because of clinical signs presumed to be related to obstruction of the urethra caused by uroliths. The owner had observed the dog unsuccessfully straining to void urine for the past 24 hours. Survey and contrast radiography confirmed the presence of numerous uroliths in the lumen of the urethra and urinary bladder (**Fig. 1**). Using retrograde urohydropropulsion, the urethroliths were returned to the urinary bladder by the emergency staff. The dog was not azotemic. Because of the large number of uroliths present in the urinary bladder, the veterinarian persuaded the client that surgery was the optimum method of removing all of the uroliths and a cystotomy was performed 12 days later. More than 100 green-colored smooth uroliths were removed (**Fig. 2**). Quantitative analysis of the uroliths at the Minnesota Urolith Center revealed that they were composed of 100% ammonium urate.

At the time the dog was released from the hospital, the owner was advised that a management protocol designed to minimize risk factors associated with ammonium urate uroliths should be seriously considered. This encompassed using a high-moisture diet designed to restrict purines and to promote formation of dilute alkaline urine

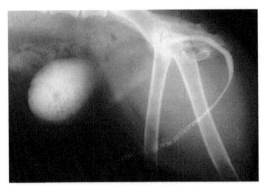

Fig. 1. Retrograde positive contrast urethrocystogram of a 4-year-old male Dalmatian illustrating numerous uroliths in the bladder and urethra.

(Prescription Diet canine u/d canned, Hill's Pet Nutrition). In addition, allopurinol was recommended.

The primary care veterinarian referred the owner to the Minnesota Urolith Center for possible enrollment in a clinical trial consisting of dietary therapy to minimize the recurrence of uroliths in Dalmatians. Twelve days following the cystotomy, the dog was admitted to the University of Minnesota Veterinary Medical Center for follow-up evaluation. According to the owner, the dog was pollakiuric for the first week following surgery. For the past 2 to 3 days he was also dysuric. Palpation of the dog's urethra revealed at least two urethroliths causing partial urethral outflow obstruction. Follow-up contrast radiography confirmed that three uroliths were present in the urethra. Because the uroliths were smooth, they were readily repulsed into the urinary bladder by retrograde urohydropropulsion. Double contrast cystography revealed that three uroliths were in the bladder lumen at that time (see **Fig. 3**). The three uroliths were approximately 0.5 cm in diameter. This prompted the owners to ask whether or not the stones had reformed during the 12-day postsurgical interval. Unfortunately, postoperative radiographs at the primary care veterinary practice were not exposed, processed, or evaluated immediately following the cystotomy to determine if all of the stones had been removed by surgery. However, the likelihood of three ammonium urate uroliths of that size forming in 12 days is highly improbable. In the authors' opinion,

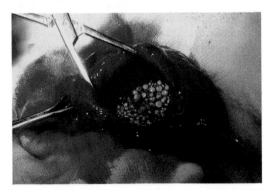

Fig. 2. More than 100 ammonium urate urocystoliths in the urinary bladder of the Dalmatian described in **Fig. 6**.

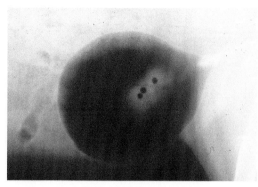

Fig. 3. Double contrast cystogram of the dog described in **Fig. 1**. There are three uroliths in the bladder lumen.

all of the uroliths were not removed by cystotomy, or the urethra was not evaluated to assure there were no urethroliths present (eg, an iatrogenic event).

When and How Should the Referring Veterinarian Be Informed of the Situation?

Following the basic admonition of the Golden Rule, the primary care veterinarian who referred the case was contacted by phone immediately. She was asked whether or not her client had been informed of the risk of not removing all of the uroliths, and the availability of some sort of postoperative imaging to evaluate her patient for this possibility. She explained that this possibility had not been considered because she had not experienced this problem previously. After further discussion, she indicated that the owner should be offered the opportunity to return to her practice for follow-up care, or remain under he care of clinicians at the Minnesota Urolith Center. With either choice, she wanted the client to know that she would absorb all expenses related to Jake's follow-up care. She would also be in direct contact with her client as soon as a time convenient to this client could be arranged. Is this the right ethical and legal choice for her to make?

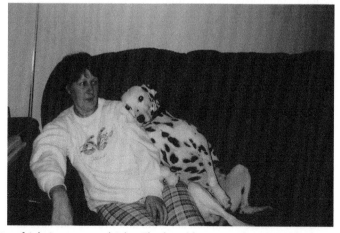

Fig. 4. Photo of Jake's owner and Jake. The bond between them is evident.

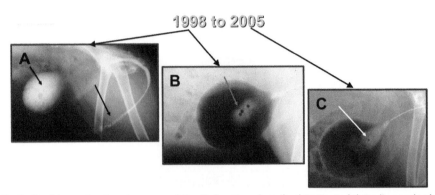

Fig. 5. Double contrast cystograms of the Dalmatian described in **Fig. 1**. (*A*) Radiograph obtained at the time when Jake was first evaluated. (*B*) Radiograph obtained following cystotomy. Three uroliths remain in the bladder lumen. (*C*) Radiograph obtained 7 years following the radiograph described in (*A*). Only one small (approximately 1 mm) urolith is present.

What Should the Owner Be Told?

The principles of veterinary medical ethics of the AVMA states in part that veterinarians should be honest and fair in their relations with others, just as they would like others to be fair and honest with them.[11] It follows that veterinarians should avoid engaging in fraud, misrepresentation, or deceit. Therefore, when a veterinarian makes mistakes caring for patients that results in significant and potentially expensive complications, or become aware of such an event, ethical conduct requires that clients be informed of this situation in a timely fashion.

Who Should Tell the Client that a Mistake Was Made?

The referring doctor was asked, "Would you like to explain this situation to your client, or would you prefer to have us provide an explanation?" After thoroughly conversing with the referring colleague, the authors informed the client of the current situation, the short-term and long-term prognosis associated with the uroliths, and the options available for management at this time. This responsibility was not delegated to lay staff; rather, the authors discussed the iatrogenic event in a private setting that fostered face-to-face communication. In situations like this one, good communication

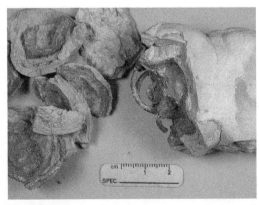

Fig. 6. Fragments of a mixture of ammonium urate and struvite that have formed around a catheter found in the bladder.

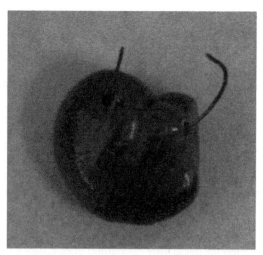

Fig. 7. Calcium oxalate monohydrate that has formed around suture material.

by all concerned individuals is essential. Why? It is the authors' opinion that good communication cannot occur without understanding, and understanding is unlikely to occur without good communication. Therefore, the authors explained in simple terms the facts related to the care provided. It was pointed out that uroliths escape detection by even the most experienced surgeons (including Board-certified surgeons). Therefore, it was emphasized that postoperative imaging is important to detect any remaining stones. This procedure is now a standard of practice.[11]

Communication about potential harm resulting from a medical mistake should be made with tact, including a compassionate expression of regret. Although not the situation in this instance, compassionately acknowledging that an untoward event has occurred need not represent an admission of responsibility. However, to the extent that is possible, the owner should be assured that efforts will be made to prevent similar events in the future. This requires a paradigm shift on the part of some veterinarians and some insurance companies.

In the authors' opinion, candid and timely disclosure of this error helped this client understand the situation and in this way enhanced her trust in all who were a part of Jake's

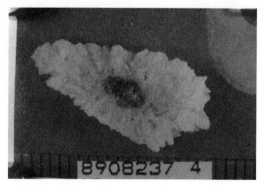

Fig. 8. Cross section of feline compound urocystolith comprised of a nidus of urate and a shell of struvite.

care. On the other hand, if iatrogenic complications are deliberately ignored or unethically disguised by dishonesty and falsification of medical records, clients who discover this deception will lose their trust in veterinarians. Deception may also motivate clients to pursue litigation.

Who Should Be Responsible for the Costs of Managing the Three Remaining Urocystoliths?

Veterinarians may also consider whether there should be an offer of restitution of expenses associated with the iatrogenic event. In this situation, consultation with the professional liability firm of which a veterinarian is a member is recommended. In Jake's example, informed consent of the client before proceeding with surgery based on knowledge of the fact that uroliths often remain following surgery, and the need to detect them by appropriate postoperative imaging techniques, might have changed the client's selection of options for therapy. Fortunately, the explanations of how this predicament developed were well received by Jake's owners. These clients were very understanding and expressed a very complimentary opinion of their primary care veterinarian for being very concerned about Jake's well-being, and for her straight-forward honesty (**Fig. 4**).

The authors were able to help resolve the question of fees by enrolling Jake in the authors' clinical trial. He remained a compliant patient in the trial for 7 years. During that time, he did not develop any new uroliths, nor was there any growth in the three existing urocystoliths. In fact, two stones either dissolved or were spontaneously voided (**Fig. 5**). During the 7-year period of study, Jake's urocystoliths remained asymptomatic.

How Could This Type of Problem Be Minimized in the Future?

The word "iatrogenic" is not synonymous with the word "malpractice." To emphasize this point, consider the following illustration. In an article written in the February 1, 1999 issue of *The New Yorker* magazine entitled, "When Doctors Make Mistakes," the byline was, "The real problem isn't how to stop bad doctors from harming, even killing, their patients. It's how to prevent good doctors from doing so."[12] The central

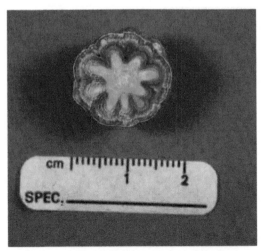

Fig. 9. Cross section of a laminated urolith comprised of a nidus of silica and a shell of struvite.

theme of this article embodied the premise that any health care provider, no matter how experienced or skilled he or she may be, could unintentionally cause harm to their patients. Could one agree that iatrogenic events are not limited to "dangerous" doctors? All participants in the veterinary profession, including highly competent and skilled specialists, cause them. Likely, those reading (and certainly the ones writing) this article have made iatrogenic errors in their efforts to provide care for their patients.

The question is, what should we as individuals—and as a profession—do about this problem? In the authors' opinion, the solution does not lie in concentrating our efforts to assess blame and shame by issuing fines or in revoking or restricting the licenses of veterinarians who make mistakes. Such an adversarial approach promotes defensiveness, secrecy, and an unwillingness to share mistakes with colleagues with the goal of understanding and preventing them.

A well-defined problem is half solved. Therefore, the first step should encompass practical mechanisms to detect, define, monitor and record the underlying events related to iatrogenic diseases, including errors of omission and errors of commission. The goal should be to fix the fault and not the blame. Once the magnitude and nature of related events are identified, procedures should be developed to eliminate or at least minimize them.

How might this apply to cats and dogs with urolithiasis? The first step is to define how frequently cystotomy is associated with incomplete removal of uroliths. In this context, a retrospective study of cystotomies performed to remove uroliths from 37 dogs and 29 cats at the University of Minnesota Veterinary Medical Center revealed incomplete removal in eight dogs and four cats.[13] The observation that uroliths were detected in the lower urinary tract following cystotomy in 20% of cats and 14% of dogs in a teaching hospital with Board-certified surgeons on the staff emphasizes an inherent risk associated with this procedure. To minimize this complication, the following procedure was developed.

When discussing the option of surgery to remove uroliths from the lower or upper urinary tract, clients should be informed that even in the hands of experienced surgeons, there is a risk that not all of the uroliths will be removed. Therefore, if the number of uroliths are such that an accurate count of each one is not feasible, appropriate radiographs will be evaluated following surgery to insure that all of them have been removed. Clients should also be informed of the consequences of incomplete removal of uroliths, and the benefits and risks of therapeutic strategies available to manage this complication.

Uroliths often migrate to lower portions of the urinary tract. Therefore, if several days have elapsed between the date of diagnostic radiography and ultrasonography and the date of surgery scheduled to remove the uroliths, the number and location of stones should be re-evaluated by appropriate imaging methods just before surgery.

Appropriate caution should be taken to remove all uroliths from the bladder lumen, bladder neck, urethra, kidneys, and ureters. When possible, the number of uroliths removed from the urinary tract should be compared with the number of uroliths detected by radiography, ultrasonography, or via uroscopy. Uroliths may be removed from different portions of the urinary tract with the aid of spoons, forceps, gauze sponges, suction devices, or stone baskets. When possible, the lumen of the bladder and bladder neck should be explored with a sterilized gloved finger to detect remaining uroliths. In some cases, an assistant can evaluate the pelvic urethra for remaining uroliths via rectal examination. The bladder lumen or kidney pelvis should be flushed with an isotonic solution to remove subvisual uroliths. Uroliths that have passed into the urethral lumen may be flushed back into the bladder lumen by injecting appropriate quantities of physiologic saline through a catheter placed in the external urethral orifice. An assistant should occlude the external urethral orifice around the catheter to facilitate flushing migrating urethroliths back into the bladder lumen. If the distal urethra is not occluded, fluid may flow round small urethroliths without moving them into the bladder lumen; this will likely result in incomplete removal of uroliths. If retrograde flushing techniques are used to flush urethroliths into the bladder with the aid of a catheter inserted into the distal urethral orifice, appropriate caution must be used to minimize retrograde flushing of bacteria that normally colonize the mucosa of the distal urethra and genital tract into the urinary bladder and surgical site. Inserting a flexible catheter through its lumen via the urinary bladder may also promote patency of the urethra. Injection of an isotonic solution through the catheter may propel uroliths out the distal urethral orifice. Appropriate precaution should be used to avoid contamination of the surgical site. In similar fashion, small nephroliths or fragments of nephroliths that have migrated into the ureters during surgery may be flushed back into the renal pelvis by retrograde flush via the ureters.

Re-evaluate appropriate radiographs of the urinary tract obtained immediately following surgery, especially when multiple uroliths are detected before cystotomy. Immediate detection of uroliths that were inadvertently left in the urinary tract is of great importance. If uroliths obstruct the urethra before the cystotomy incision heals, life-threatening complications may develop. Furthermore, if uroliths remaining in the lower urinary tract following surgery are not detected by radiography or ultrasonography until several weeks following surgery, it may be erroneously assumed that the patient is highly predisposed to recurrent urolithiasis. We call this phenomenon "pseudorecurrence."

Questionable Prognoses

What about diseases (such as ureteroliths) for which the risk and benefit ratios of various treatments cannot always be clearly forecast? When uncertainty exists as to whether or not a particular drug, medical, or surgical procedure is or is not in the best interests of the patient, the authors try to answer the following questions in context of the Golden Rule: Based on all information available, would I choose this course of therapy if I were this patient? Based on knowledge of my own skill and experience, and the availability of support staff and the ability to monitor therapeutic response, would I consent to the proposed plan of therapeutic action if I were in this patient's exact situation? What therapeutic goals are likely to be achieved? If I do follow the proposed plan of therapy, in all probability will the overall benefits of this plan justify the associated risks and costs?

QUANTITATIVE UROLITH ANALYSIS
A Standard of Practice

A quarter century ago, analysis of uroliths removed (usually by a surgical technique) by veterinarians was optional. In fact, rather than have the stones analyzed, some veterinary practitioners gave the uroliths to their clients as a topic of conversation. What about today? Is it an acceptable standard of practice to give stones retrieved from the urinary tract to owners without confirming their composition? What would be your response to a physician who gave you stones retrieved from your urinary tract? The question that is posed is whether making a choice not to request quantitative analysis of uroliths is ethical. Should failure to request quantitative urolith analysis be considered as negligence?

Recall that negligence may be defined as the act of doing (or not doing) something that a person of ordinary prudence would not have done (or would have done) under similar circumstances. Being negligent implies that a veterinarian did not follow a reasonable standard of care. The standard of care not only applies to what is done (commission), but also what is not done (omission). The law says that reasonable practitioners, not the most highly skilled professionals, set the standard of care. If an error occurs despite the exercise of due care, the issue of negligence is not involved. In this context, should failure to request quantitative urolith analysis be considered as negligence?

What Are Uroliths?

Uroliths are aggregates of mineral or nonmineral substances located in the urinary tract. Uroliths may vary in size and number, and may form in one or more locations within the urinary tract when urine becomes over-saturated with crystallogenic substances. Uroliths may be composed of one or more biogenic minerals, including magnesium ammonium phosphate (struvite), calcium phosphate (calcium apatite), calcium oxalate monohydrate (whewellite), calcium oxalate dihydrate (weddellite), uric acid or salts of uric acid (ammonium, sodium, and calcium urate), silica, cystine, and xanthine. They may also be partially or completely composed of drugs or drug metabolites. If foreign substances (for example, suture material, hair, or plant material such as awns) are present within the lumen of the urinary tract, they often become the nidus for urolith formation (**Figs. 6** and **7**).

Why Should Uroliths Be Analyzed?

At our current level of understanding, medical treatment and prevention of the causes underlying urolithiasis are dependent on the knowledge of the composition and structure of the entire stone. Minerals in uroliths may be deposited in distinct layers or they may be admixed throughout the stones. Although one mineral type usually predominates, the composition of uroliths is frequently mixed (for example, 90% struvite and 10% calcium phosphate). The center (nidus) may be composed of one mineral type (such as calcium oxalate), whereas outer layers may be composed of one (such as struvite) or more different mineral types (**Figs. 8** and **9**). Therefore, all uroliths retrieved from a patient should be submitted for quantitative analysis. This paradigm change is now a standard of practice in our profession.

In addition to quantitative analysis, nonsurgical methods of urolith management in cats and dogs have also become a standard of practice in the veterinary profession. Choice of treatment or prevention based on results of quantitative mineral analysis of stones consistently provides the most favorable outcome.

How can Uroliths be Retrieved for Analysis?

Until the beginning of the 1980s, surgery was considered as the only practical method of removal of uroliths. However, the authors have devised several different means to move and remove uroliths from the patient. Small urocystoliths can be retrieved from the urinary bladder by "jiggling" the stones in the bladder, while urine or saline and small stones are aspirated through a urinary catheter into a syringe.[14] Uroliths may also be removed from the urinary bladder by voiding urohydropropulsion.[15] Urocystoliths spontaneously voided through the urethral lumen to the exterior may be harvested with the aid of a small aquarium fishnet placed into the patient's urine stream. These tropical fishnets are available at most pet stores and are inexpensive. Stone baskets may also be used to remove uroliths. Additional information about these techniques of urolith removal can be obtained from the January 1999 edition of the *Veterinary Clinics of North America* under the title, "The Rocket Science of Canine Urolithiasis."[16]

Box 1
Do's and dont's of urolith submission for quantitative urolith analysis

DO NOT give uroliths obtained from a patient to owners. If it becomes necessary to give them a sample of the uroliths, wait until the composition of the uroliths is known.

DO submit uroliths for quantitative analysis.

DO NOT submit stones for qualitative analysis.

DO submit all uroliths collected from the patient or submit representative sizes and appearances if numerous uroliths are available.

DO NOT submit just one stone if many are present. Uroliths may form at different times, and at different locations in the same patient, and therefore they may vary in composition.

DO NOT submit only portions of uroliths. Small portions may not be representative of the entire urolith.

DO NOT crush or fragment uroliths because it is likely to interfere with identification and evaluation of the layers within the stone.

DO submit uroliths dry.

DO NOT submit uroliths in formalin, because formalin may change the composition of the stone.

DO consider obtaining an appropriate size of urinary bladder or kidney tissue if such samples can be safely obtained at the time of surgical or uroscopic removal of a patient's uroliths. These biopsy specimens should be placed in an appropriate fixative and saved for future use. If, at a later time there is no need for them, they may be discarded. However, if the nature of the underlying or concomitant disorder requires biopsy samples for further evaluation, the samples will be available without further need for invasive techniques.

DO accurately and completely fill out the appropriate urolith submission form. Most laboratories request the following information: owner's name, species, breed of that species, gender and reproductive status of the patient, birth date, history of medications currently or previously taken, previous episodes of uroliths and if yes, mineral type of previous uroliths.

DO package uroliths in noncrushable containers. If samples arrive at the Urolith Center crushed, different layers of minerals within a stone cannot be identified. If samples are placed in standard envelopes used for mailing sheets of paper, uroliths are often forced through the side of the mailing envelope by automated equipment used to rapidly process mail by the United States Postal Service.

DO affix sufficient postage to the package containing uroliths to ensure timely delivery to the urolith center.

DO review quantitative urolith analysis results with the goal of selecting the urolith management prescription associated with the greatest benefits and the fewest risks.

If you have questions, first consult the Web site of the Minnesota Urolith Center at www.cvm.umn.edu; Click the link to departments and centers to find the button for the Minnesota Urolith Center. Follow the menu for the following information:

About us

Before you submit samples

Contact us

Frequently asked questions

How to submit samples

How to interpret results

Recent publications

Recommendations

Urolith cultures

What to do while waiting for results.

How Should Uroliths Be Submitted for Analysis?

Methods by which uroliths are submitted for analysis may have a substantial impact on the quality of the analysis. **Box 1** shows a step-by-step list of the do's and do not's of urolith submission.

What Methods of Analysis Are Recommended?

Two general methods of urolith analysis may be considered: qualitative analysis and quantitative analysis. The misleadingly named qualitative analysis, is usually performed using spot chemical tests to identify chemical radicals and ions. This archaic method of analysis has been virtually abandoned because it is unreliable. Most qualitative techniques require pulverizing the stone for analysis; therefore, layers of different minerals frequently identified by quantitative methods of analysis typically cannot be identified. Furthermore, these tests were not designed to identify many crystalline components that occur in uroliths, including amorphous silica and silica salts, drugs, and drug metabolites (eg, sulfadiazine), newberyite, boberyite, uric acid and its salts, and others. Qualitative tests are insensitive to detection of calcium and salts of calcium. In the authors' experience, all qualitative tests for biogenic minerals are insensitive and lack specificity. They should not be used.

Several physical methods of urolith analysis allow detection and varying degrees of quantification of minerals present in stones. These methods include optical crystallography, infrared spectroscopy, X-ray diffraction, energy-dispersive techniques, and others. Optical crystallography is based on use of a polarizing microscope to identify crystalline components of uroliths (**Fig. 10**). Representative sections of the stone are identified with the aid of a dissecting microscope. These samples (or crystal grains, as they are sometimes called) are then viewed with a polarizing scope. Optical properties, such as refractive index and birefringence, characteristic of different minerals, are then recorded and compared with known standards to determine the mineral types.

Infrared spectroscopy is based on the observation that when infrared waves encounter a sample, some is absorbed by the sample (absorbance) and some passes through the sample (transmission). The resulting spectrum that is created is a molecular fingerprint of the sample (**Fig. 11**). Because no two unique molecular structures

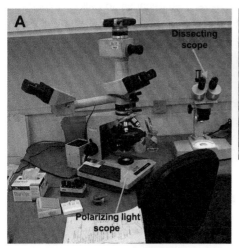
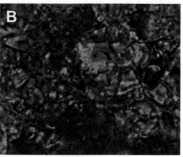

Fig. 10. (*A*) Optical crystallography is based on use of a polarizing microscope to identify crystalline components of uroliths. (*B*) Calcium oxalate monohydrate (original magnification ×450).

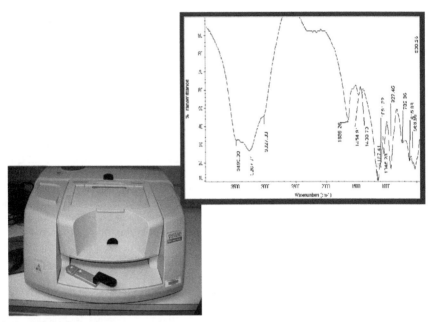

Fig. 11. Infrared spectroscopy.

produce the same infrared spectrum, these spectra can be compared with known reference spectra for identification. This procedure is very useful in accurately identifying unknown materials, determining the quality and consistency of samples, and quantifying the amounts of different calculogenic substances within the sample.

Unfortunately, some laboratories persist in performing qualitative analysis. They justify performing this archaic method by claiming that a qualitative test was ordered by the doctor caring for the patient. The implication is that veterinarians ordering the qualitative tests are aware of the limitations of these procedures, and therefore the tests are valid. Some laboratories argue that qualitative test results (even if incorrect) can provide results in less than 24 hours. However, just because so-called "experts" derive test results does not validate the test results. One technique that may provide

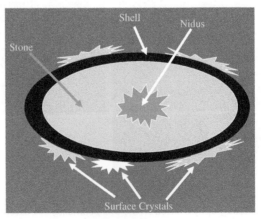

Fig. 12. Cross section of a urolith and it's various parts.

some insight into recognizing this problem is to split a urolith and send representatives portions to more than one laboratory at the same time. If the results are significantly different, this may be a cause for concern. Some of the laboratories performing qualitative urolith tests charge a fee comparable to that charged by laboratories that perform quantitative mineral analysis. It is likely that their motive for providing qualitative test results is profit. The persons responsible for allowing this disservice are not meeting the current standard of practice in the United States.

All laboratories do not report the results obtained by quantitative analysis in the same fashion. Regardless of the method of analysis, the location of minerals within the urolith should be specified (**Fig. 12**). Layers that are grossly visible by examination of cross sections of stones may or may not contain different types of minerals (see **Figs. 8** and **9**). Formation of metabolic uroliths (eg, calcium oxalate) followed by formation of infection-induced magnesium ammonium phosphate (eg, infection-induced struvite) may result in distinct laminations detected by survey radiography or by examination of the cut surface of the stone. If significant hemorrhage occurs intermittently, it may affect the appearance of layers on the cut surface without a corresponding change in the mineral composition of the urolith.

REFERENCES

1. Starr P. The Social transformations of American medicine. New York: Basic Books; 1982. p. 3–29.
2. Anonymous. Principles of veterinary medical ethics of the American Veterinary Medical Association. Schaumburg (IL): AVMA Directory; 2007. p. 36–8.
3. Wilson JF. Law and ethics of the veterinary profession. Morrisville (PA): Priority Press Ltd; 2005.
4. Seldes G. The great quotations. Secaucus (NJ): Citadel Press; 1983. p. 225, 283.
5. Osborne CA. The veterinarian's oath. Are you keeping your promise? J Am Vet Med Assoc 1991;198:1906–8.
6. Taylor EJ, editor. Dorland's Illustrated Medical Dictionary. 27th edition. Philadelphia: WB Saunders; 1988. p. 812, iatrogenic; page 1361, prognosis.
7. Guyatt G, Cairns J, Churchill D, et al. Evidence-Based Medicine Working Group. Evidence-based medicine. A new approach to teaching the practice of medicine. J Am Med Assoc 1992;268:2420–5.
8. Sackett DL, Rosenberg WM, Gray JA. Evidence based medicine. What it is, and what it isn't. BMJ 1996;312:71–2.
9. Strauss MB. Familiar medical quotations. Boston: Little, Brown & Co.; 1968. p 49.
10. Osborne CA. Don't just do something, stand there. An exposition of hippocrates admonition, first do no harm. Compendium on Continuing Education for the Practicing Veterinarian 1991;13(8):1248–62.
11. Anonymous. Omission of radiograph falls below standard of care. Professional liability insurance trust. American Veterinary Medical Association 2005;24(3):1–2.
12. Gawande A. When doctors make mistakes. New Yorker Magazine 1999;41–55.
13. Lulich J, Osborne C, Polzin D, et al. Incomplete removal of canine and feline urocystoliths by cystotomy. J Vet Intern Med 1993;7:124.
14. Osborne CA, Lulich JP, Polzin DJ. Canine retrograde urohydropulsion: lessons from 25 years of experience. Vet Clin North Am 1999;29:267–82.
15. Lulich JP, Osborne CA, Sanderson SL, et al. Voiding urohydropulsion: lessons from 5 years of experience. Vet Clin North Am 1991;29:267–91.
16. Osborne CA, Lulich JP, Bartges JW. The rocket science of canine urolithiasis. Vet Clin North Am 1999;29:1–306.

Changing Paradigms in Diagnosis of Inherited Defects Associated with Urolithiasis

Danika Bannasch, DVM, PhD[a,b,*], Paula S. Henthorn, PhD[c]

KEYWORDS

- Genetic • Gene • Urate • Hyperuricosuria
- Cystinuria • Cystine

CANINE GENOMICS

A dog genome sequence was made publicly available in 2004 and is the basis of a new paradigm in the study, diagnosis, and treatment of inherited diseases in dogs. In reality, the way in which veterinary scientists think about and approach the study of genetic disease has not changed, but the tools available to veterinary scientists have and will continue to change, allowing us to study increasingly complex problems and to make more rapid advances in the context of simple problems. To put these advances in perspective, this article first gives a historical perspective on the approaches to studying genetic diseases, particularly in human beings, and then outlines the advances that have become possible with the availability of the dog genome sequence. The article then discusses two inherited defects that are associated with urolithiasis, in particular: those responsible for cystine and purine (uric acid and its salts) stone formation. Together, these two conditions illustrate the contemporary use of a broad range of genetic approaches.

No matter what species are investigated, geneticists base their approach to the study of a disease on the information available about that disease. The information falls into two broad categories: one category encompasses what is known at the

This work was supported by grants from the National Institute of Health (NIDDK DK074954 and RR02512), and grants from the Morris Animal Foundation and the Canine Health Foundation.

[a] Department of Population Health and Reproduction, School of Veterinary Medicine, One Shields Avenue, University of California, Davis, Davis, CA 95616, USA

[b] Veterinary Medical Teaching Hospital, School of Veterinary Medicine, University of California, Davis, Davis, CA, USA

[c] Department of Clinical Studies-Philadelphia, School of Veterinary Medicine, 3900 Delancey Street, University of Pennsylvania, Philadelphia, PA 19104-6010, USA

* Corresponding author. Department of Population Health and Reproduction, School of Veterinary Medicine, One Shields Avenue, University of California, Davis, Davis, CA 95616, USA.

E-mail address: dlbannasch@ucdavis.edu (D. Bannasch).

protein, cellular, organ, and whole organism level; the second category encompasses what is known at the DNA level. Using these terms loosely, one can think of the information as based either on the phenotype or the genome category. Phenotypic information can consist of specific enzyme activity or results of any specific laboratory or clinical assay, whereas the genomic category may include information about anatomy, development, behavior, or abnormalities of a cell type, organ, or the entire living being. Genomic information can range from understanding of the mode of inheritance through the study of families in which the disease is found, the description of a chromosomal abnormality, or any knowledge of the location of the DNA sequence variation that is responsible for a disease or other nondeleterious phenotypic characteristic. Information about a particular companion animal disease should also take into account what is known about similar diseases in other species, particularly in other mammals, such as human beings and mice.

Most of the initial studies that identified DNA mutations underlying genetic disease were based on phenotypic knowledge of the defective, absent, or inappropriate protein, abnormally expressed in a human disease. Through time-consuming and laborious methods, the cDNAs (complementary DNA, also called "copy DNA"; cDNA is DNA produced by reverse transcriptase acting on messenger RNA) and genes for these proteins were cloned and sequenced from affected and normal individuals, leading to the discovery of disease-causing DNA mutations. This knowledge spilled over into veterinary medicine, leading to identification of underlying disease-causing mutations for diseases such as hemophilia, lysosomal storage diseases, and other simple inherited diseases caused by enzyme deficiencies. For example, canine phosphofructokinase deficiency and mucopolysaccharidosis (MPS) VII were understood at the molecular level in this fashion.[1,2] In these cases, the absence of a particular protein or enzyme activity indicated which genes might be defective. Prior cloning of these genes in humans or other mammals provided information and reagents that allowed their study in companion animals. In other words, the early approaches to understanding the DNA basis of genetic diseases, including the choice of genes that could be considered as candidate-genes to study, were based entirely on phenotypic information about the diseases and their pathology.

In the 1980s, the approach to study of genetic disease based on genome position began to be used and is now generally referred to as "positional cloning." This approach initially used a combination of cytogenetic data (ie, observations of deletions of particular parts of chromosomes in affected individuals) and genetic mapping data. Genetic mapping refers to analyzing polymorphic sites (places in the genome where the DNA is known to vary in sequence between different individuals in the species) in families that contain one or more individuals affected with the disease of interest. The goal is to identify sites of DNA variation at variant alleles (alleles are different forms or variants of a gene found at the same place—or locus—on a chromosome) that travel from generation to generation with the disease. Various manifestations of the disease occur when the site of DNA variation is located on the same chromosome and close to the gene and mutation that causes disease. Consequently, by knowing the chromosomal location of the variable DNA sequence (also known as a "linked-marker"), one can detemine the approximate location of a disease-causing gene. The next step is to search the DNA surrounding the linked marker for the disease-causing gene and mutation. At one time, this was extremely time consuming. Fortunately, recent advances, including the development of polymerase chain reaction technology, the availability of whole genome sequences, and some other genomic tools have considerably simplified the last steps involved in positional cloning.

What Is a Genome Sequence and How Is It Used?

A genome sequence is the complete DNA sequence of all of the chromosomes of a particular living being (except the Y chromosome in some cases). For mammalian species, a genome sequence is comprised of between 2.4 and 3 billion nucleotides. Genome sequences are currently generated by isolating genomic DNA from the organism of interest and breaking or cutting the chromosome-length DNA molecules into predetermined sizes that can be readily cloned and sequenced. Once the sequencing of the ends of millions of clones has been completed, a super computer is used to (1) compare the sequences to one another to identify overlapping sequences; (2) organize the individual sequences; and (3) determine the consensus sequence of each chromosome. If more DNA is sequenced, each individual base is sequenced more frequently and the resulting genome sequence is likely to be more accurate. For the dog genome sequence, over 31 million sequences were generated (each dataset consisting of between 500 and 600 nucleotides, on average) and resulted in assemble-genome sequences where each nucleotide was sequenced an average of 7.6 times. This is referred to as a "7.6 X genome sequence" and represents 99% of the dog genome.

Other sequence-based resources include databases of expressed sequence tags (ESTs). ESTs are generated from cloning all mRNA molecules from particular tissues or cell types, then sequencing the ends of these clones in effort to capture all of the mRNA molecules made by a particular being. If exhaustively cloned and analyzed, these mRNA molecules define all of the possible protein sequences encoded by the DNA of a particular species. When aligned to a whole genome sequence to show regions of identical DNA sequence, they pinpoint the location of the gene that encodes the mRNA and protein.

Other extremely useful DNA sequences are those that are variable within a species, (also known as polymorphisms). Databases exist that annotate all known single-nucleotide polymorphisms (SNPs). This type of variation is particularly useful because high-through-put assays have been developed (also called "SNP chips") that can determine the alleles present at hundreds of thousands of SNPs of an individual in a single experiment. The dog genome-sequencing project identified more than 2.5 million SNPs. In addition, the technology now exists to simultaneously analyze more than 120,000 dog SNPs.

With so much DNA sequence information, the only practical method of interpreting and annotating the sequences is via a computer. Several genome browsers have been developed that are extremely helpful in integrating available DNA sequence data, with graphical interfaces that identify the location of gene, mRNAs, ESTs, SNPs, and evolutionarily conserved sequences that reside along the linear length of the chromosome. There are three main genome browsers available for the dog, the National Center for Biotechnology Information (www.ncbi.nlm.nih.gov/genome/guide/dog), the Santa Cruz Genome browser (genome.ucsc.edu), and Ensembl (www.ensembl.org/index.html).

How Will Availability of Genome Sequences, and Other Sequence-Based Information and Technologies Change the Way Genetic Diseases Can Be Studied in the Future?

Knowledge of as much about the phenotype of the disease as possible will still be of the utmost importance. As this article explains, technologically advanced genetic studies will remain of limited use if disease phenotypes are not well defined with appropriate information available for affected and unaffected animals. Family studies will still be relevant, as this information will continue to be useful in predicting the mode of inheritance of a particular disease or trait and also to identify breeds that are at increased risk for a particular disease. However, genome sequences and related technologies are accelerating the rate at which discoveries are made and confirmed, and allow the study of diseases that are more complex in their inheritance (eg, susceptibility to cancer and autoimmunity), compared with those which are simple inherited diseases.

The current approach to a complex genetic disease is based on the assumption that, particularly within a breed, the disease is caused by the same DNA mutation that was inherited from a common ancestor to all affected dogs. Therefore, all affected dogs share at least the part of the ancestral chromosome that contains the gene that suffered the disease-causing mutation. They will also share some amount of DNA surrounding that gene, and that DNA will in essence be "marked" by the particular pattern of DNA variation that was present in the ancestor dog. For some diseases, the original disease-causing mutation may have occurred before the breed was formed, so that today the same mutation occurs in different breeds. Based on these assumptions, the current approach to a genetic disease will typically proceed in the manner described in the following example.

A disease is recognized as having a genetic basis because it has a particularly high incidence in one breed and a somewhat high incidence in several breeds, while multiple breeds also appear to be protected from the disease. In high incidence breeds, there have been reports of litters with multiple affected offspring, but there have been enough investigations of the disease to demonstrate that parent-to-offspring transmission is a rare event. This information leads to the conclusion that the disease does not show simple autosomal dominant transmission and that the disease occurs with equal frequency in males and females. DNA is collected from affected dogs in the high-risk breed, as well as unaffected dogs of the same breed that have been thoroughly examined and, when possible, are older than the age at which the disease is usually diagnosed. Appropriate evaluations have proved that they do not have the disease. The DNA sample from each dog of this group is analyzed to determine the location of alleles (genotype) at tens of thousands of SNPs across the dog genome, using available high-throughput technologies such as "SNP chips" (currently both Affymetrix and Illumina offer canine SNP arrays). The massive amount of data that is obtained is statistically analyzed to identify SNPs at which the allele frequencies vary significantly between the affected dogs (cases) and the unaffected dogs (controls). An example would be the extreme case where, at a particular SNP, all affected dogs have an adenosine nucleotide (A) on both copies of the chromosome, while all the control dogs are either heterozygous for A and C (cytosine) or homozygous for C. The assumption in this example is that the association of the A allele with the disease phenotype is because of the original disease-causing mutation that occurred nearby on the chromosome that contained an A allele at this particular SNP. It has traveled with the disease-causing mutation through the generations that have passed since the mutation occurred. Because the location of the SNP is known, the next step is to look at the dog genome sequence in the region of the SNP, determining what genes are nearby, and finding out what is known about the function and expression of those genes. If it seems possible that the genes could be involved in the disease, they are then considered as candidate genes. Candidate genes are then sequenced in normal and affected dogs to determine if there are any DNA differences that might account for the disease. If so, additional experiments can be designed to prove that the DNA difference is actually the cause of the disease. Once candidate genes have been identified, much of what is known about a gene is likely to be information obtained from the study of humans and mice.

Once a disease-causing mutation has been identified, the potential benefits are both immediate and long term. Of immediate benefit is the ability to use the knowledge of the specific disease-causing DNA change for genetic testing, to provide information needed to reduce the incidence of the particular genetic disease. Of long-term benefit is the possibility that the knowledge of the molecular basis of the disease will lead to new therapies that could range from the development of a new pharmacologic agent to the administration of a DNA-based (gene-) or cell-based (stem cell) therapy.

GENETIC BASIS FOR UROLITHIASIS IN DOGS

Certain types of uroliths are more likely to have a genetic basis than others. Primary changes in metabolism that lead to increased urine concentration of compounds that can form uroliths are the most obvious inherited causes of urolithiasis. In dogs, both cystine and uric acid can be excreted in urine in increased quantities because of metabolic changes resulting in cystinuria or hyperuricosuria. Some of the genes responsible for these disorders have been identified. In both of these cases, the metabolic change that leads to abnormally high concentrations of uric acid or cystine results in an increased risk for urolith formation.

In addition to these primary causes, predisposing factors exist that could have a genetic basis. For example, genetic factors that predispose dogs to urinary tract infections could increase the prevalence of infection-induced struvite uroliths. Another example is studies evaluating breed associations with specific types of uroliths.[3] These studies have provided some evidence that struvite urolithiasis occurs in some particular breeds more than in others. In particular, breeds with a male predisposition to struvite urolithiasis (Cocker spaniels, Springer spaniels, and Labrador retrievers) have the potential to harbor a susceptibility locus because infection-induced struvite uroliths are generally less common in male dogs.

Urinary inhibitors and promoters of uroliths have been observed in the urine of humans and several other species, including dogs.[4,5] Genetic changes that lead to variation in the concentrations of these compounds in the urine could lead to increased risk for urolithaisis.[6] General susceptibility to urolithiasis could also occur because of inherited anatomic differences of dogs. For example, the dependency of an individual dog's bladder could lead to a predisposition to urethral obstruction. Anytime there is a breed predisposition to a particular urolith type, there is probably an underlying genetic factor that affects the prevalence in that breed.

HYPERURICOSURIA

Hyperuricosuria is defined as abnormal increase in the concentration of uric acid in the urine. Comparison of the excretion or concentration of urine uric acid in Dalmatians to some (but by no means all) different types of dogs revealed that when specific and sensitive methodology for quantification of urine uric acid was used, all the Dalmatians had hyperuricosuria.[7] Normal concentration of uric acid in dogs with normal renal function is considered to be low at approximately 9.5 mg/dL.[8] Humans excrete about 3.5 times this quantity because of a defect in the enzyme uricase (also known as uric acid oxidase) that converts uric acid to allantoin in the liver.[9] Allantoin is the end product of DNA and RNA metabolism in dogs and is much more soluble in urine than uric acid. In addition to hyperuricosuria, humans have hyperuricemia (high-serum concentrations of uric acid). **Table 1** summarizes the relative amounts of serum and urine uric acid in dogs and humans. These values do not reflect the body weights of the different species, which would make the canine numbers even higher. Humans suffer from consequences of elevated serum uric acid, including gout, which is caused by precipitation of uric acid

Table 1
Relative amounts of uric acid in serum and urine in dogs and people

Mg/dl	Human	Dog[a]	Dalmatian[a]
Serum uric acid	5-6	0.5	1.3
Urine uric acid	~33.3	~9.5	~37.8

[a] Values in mg/100 mL, converted from Moulin and colleagues.[8]

in the joints. Dalmatians with mild increases of serum uric acid do not develop signs typical of gout (see **Table 1**).

In dogs, excessive urinary excretion of uric acid can occur secondary to metabolic defects or because of particular disease states, including generalized liver disease and portosystemic shunts. The enzyme urate oxidase appears to be exclusively produced in the liver. Consequently, severe liver disease can lead to a reduced quantity of uricase and varying degrees of hyperuricemia.[10] In human beings, tumor lysis syndrome leads to excess uric acid in serum and subsequently in urine; however, this syndrome has not been documented in dogs. The biochemical pathway of purine degradation is shown in **Fig. 1**. Decreased quantities of urate oxidase leads to hyperuricemia in humans and great apes. The same phenotype can be seen in dogs with severe liver damage or port-systemic shunts.

Metabolic hyperuricosuria has been extensively studied in the Dalmatian breed of dog. There is a consensus of opinion that all Dalmatians are affected by this disorder.[7,11] In these dogs, the defect is not in the enzyme urate oxidase as it is in humans, although on the surface the phenotypes appear similar.[12] In contrast to humans, Dalmatians excrete more uric acid into the urine, resulting in lower serum uric acid concentrations than occurs in humans.

Normally, uric acid is filtered by glomerului and then reabsorbed by the proximal tubules, where it re-enters circulation. There are species-specific differences in relative amounts of reabsorption and secretion of uric acid by the proximal tubules.[13] The proteins involved in the reabsorption of uric acid from the ultrafiltrate are just beginning to be discovered. Uric acid must be transported across the apical membrane of the proximal tubules and then across the basolateral membrane in order to re-enter the systemic circulation. Micropuncture experiments were used to demonstrate that there is a reduction of proximal tubular reabsorption of uric acid in Dalmatian kidneys.[14]

Based on studies that localized the Dalmatian defect to the liver,[15] Giesecke and Tiemeyer[16] studied the biochemical function of the enzyme uric acid oxidase. These investigators demonstrated that while uric acid oxidase functions in non-Dalmatian liver homogenates and liver slices, Dalmatian uric acid oxidase was only able to convert uric acid to allantoin in liver homogenates and not in liver slices. On the basis of these observations, it was suggested that the Dalmatian phenotype could be explained by the lack of function of a urate transporter in the liver.[16–18]

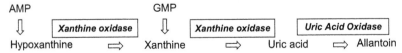

Fig. 1. Biochemical steps in the degradation of purines (enzymes that catalyze the reactions are boxed). *Abbreviations:* AMP, adenine monophosphate; GMP, guanine monophosphate.

Because the Dalmatian phenotype involves liver metabolism and urinary excretion of uric acid, investigators studied liver and kidney tissues to determine the organ responsible for the problem. The hyperuricosuria defect was localized to the liver of affected dogs by transplantation studies. It is possible to correct the defect in Dalmatians and induce hyperuricosuria in wild-type dogs by transplanting the liver or hepatocytes between Dalmatian and non-Dalmatian dogs.[15] When similar studies were done with kidney transplants, the affected phenotype could be improved but not corrected completely.[19] Based on these observations, it is currently the general consensus of opinion that hyperuricosuria is caused by a kidney phenotype and a liver phenotype in the Dalmatian and is associated with a defect in a uric acid transporter in both tissues.

Based on the outcomes of experimental crosses between a few different breeds and Dalmatians, Dalmatian hyperuricosuria is thought to be inherited as a simple autosomal recessive trait.[11,20] Clinical manifestations of this change in urinary metabolism are estimated to occur in about 25% of male Dalmatians.[21] The clinical outcome of hyperuricosuria in the Dalmatian is apparently limited to urate uroliths. Ammonium urate uroliths and uroliths composed of other salts of uric acid are much less frequently observed in female Dalmatians as compared with male Dalmatians.[22]

Because all Dalmatians are apparently affected with hyperuricosuria, cross breeding is necessary to identify the gene and the mutation that causes hyperuricosuria. To maintain the breed characteristics of the Dalmatian, Dr. Robert Schaible performed a Dalmatian-by-Pointer × Dalmatian backcross to segregate offspring into two groups: a low urine uric acid group and a high urine uric acid group. To determine if offspring excreted high or low concentrations of uric acid, puppies from this backcross were tested for urine uric acid/creatinine values when they were 4 to 7 weeks of age. **Fig. 2** shows a comparison of urine uric acid/creatinine values for pure Dalmatians, non-Dalmatians, and two classes of backcross dogs (low urine uric acid and high urine uric acid).

To map the hyperuricosuria locus, a set of markers were used to scan the canine chromosomes and identify a region that was inherited along with uric acid levels. A total of 148 markers were genotyped on 25 members of the backcross family. A single marker on chromosome CFA03, REN153P03, revealed linkage to the phenotype with a significant logarithm of the odds (LOD) score of 3.99. Additional markers from the region were tested on 36 family members and a maximum LOD score of 6.55 was obtained for REN153P03.[23] Additional markers tested in this family localized the critical interval containing the gene to a small region of the genome containing 19 candidate genes.

Because all Dalmatians are homozygous for the hyperuricosuria locus, the next approach was to identify the region of the chromosome where the DNA is identical in all Dalmatians. This further narrowed the list of genes to four candidates. Sequence analysis revealed a mutation in one gene that completely segregated with high uric acid status in the backcross dogs and was homozygous in 200 unrelated Dalmatians. The mutation was not detected in 300 non-Dalmatians.[24]

Other breeds have been reported to have a higher-than-expected incidence of urate stones, including the Bulldog and the Black Russian terrier.[3,25] When the authors tested dogs from these two breeds that had formed urate uroliths, the tests revealed the dogs were also homozygous for the mutation. Because there is no known direct relationship between the Dalmatian, Bulldog, and Black Russian terrier, the authors believe that this mutation is very old and likely to occur in other breeds as well. In the Bulldog and Black Russian terrier, the mutation segregates within the breeds, allowing breeders to use genetic testing of the mutation to select

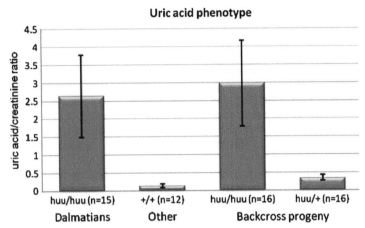

Fig. 2. Uric Acid/creatinine ratios were measured on 4- to 6-week-old puppies from the breeds shown in the figure. The animal's genotype at the hyperuricosuria locus (huu) and the number of animals sampled in each column shown is shown below each bar. Statistically significant differences were obtained by ANOVA between the +/+, huu/+, and huu/huu categories ($P = 8.33 \times 10^{-13}$, alpha 0.05). In addition, there was no difference between the two huu/huu categories (Dalmatian vs. backcross).

against hyperuricosuria. In the Dalmatian breed, the only way to eliminate hyperuricosuria, and therefore the predisposition to form urate uroliths, is by using the low uric acid backcross dogs (99.6% Dalmatian) in breeding programs. Currently, the United Kennel Club, the second largest purebred dog registry in the United States, allows these animals to be registered and therefore alter the prevalence of hyperuricoruia in the breed. At the time of writing this article, these dogs were not registered with the American Kennel Club, the largest registry in the United States, because of a decision made by the parent club for the breed, the Dalmatian Club of America. Although breed purity is important in purebred dogs, the small amount of Pointer DNA remaining in these dogs (<0.05%) seems a small price to pay for disease elimination.

CYSTINURIA

Cystinuria is a disorder of transmembrane transport of the sulfur-containing nonessential amino acid cystine and dibasic amino acids lysine, ornithine, and arginine, which normally occur in renal tubule cells after glomerular filtration and also in the intestine. Clinical manifestations result from impaired reabsorption of cystine from glomerular filtrate, leading to excess cystine in the urine. Cystine, but not the dibasic amino acids, has low solubility in acidic urine, with only small elevations above the normal concentration exceeding the acid urine saturation point.[26] As a result of cystinuria, affected humans and animals are at increased risk for formation of cystine uroliths. The impaired intestinal absorption of these four amino acids does not appear to lead to any nutritional deficiency states in dogs or humans, presumably because they are nonessential amino acids.[27]

Development of a cystine urolith in a dog was first recognized in 1823, and the first documented case of cystinuria in a dog with evidence of a metabolic defect (elevated cystine levels in the urine accompanied by urolith formation) appeared in 1935.[28,29]

Recognition of the heritable nature of cystine stone formation in dogs soon followed when Green and colleagues'[30] reported the disease in Irish terriers. Increased risk for cystine urolith formation has subsequently been documented for many breeds (summarized below).

Cystinuria has been recognized in humans for even longer than it has been documented in dogs, with discoveries in humans influencing studies in dogs. Cystinuria is recognized in two forms in humans: type I and non-type I. Type I refers to cases that show recessive inheritance and in which carriers have normal urinary amino acid concentrations. In non-type I cystinuria, the parents of patients show moderately elevated urine concentratons of cystine and the dibasic amino acids, lysine, arginine, and ornithine, and have a low incidence of cystine urolith formation. This genetic pattern is described as autosomal dominant inheritance with incomplete penetrance based on the rare incidence of cystine urolith formation in obligate carrier individuals.[27]

The molecular basis for cystinuria in humans is well documented, beginning with the first discovery of mutations in human patients.[31] It is now known that mutations in two different genes account for the disease state in greater than 95% of human patients.[32] These two genes, SLC3A1 and SLC7A9, encode the polypeptide subunits of the $b^{0,+}$ amino acid transporter (for reviews, see[27,33,34]). The system $b^{0,+}$ amino acid transport is one of several known heteromeric amino acid transporters, which are composed of a heavy chain of the SLC3 (solute carrier family 3) family, and a light chain of the SLC7 family. The SLC7 subunits, composed of 12 transmembrane domains, provide the specific amino acid transport activity and are linked to the heavy subunit by a single disulfide bond. The SLC3 subunits have a single transmembrane domain with a cytoplasmic amino terminus. The majority of this heavy chain is extracellular and heavily glycosylated. The SLC3 heavy chain appears to be essential for localization of the heteromeric transporter to the plasma membrane.[34]

The defective genes in human cystinuria are SLC3A1, encoding a protein called rBAT, and SLC7A9, encoding the protein referred to as $b^{0,+}$ AT. Over 170 different mutations in these two genes have been identified in cystinuric human patients.[32] With only one exception,[35] all of the SLC3A1 mutations are associated with type I cystinuria. In SLC7A9, nearly 85% of the SLC7A9 mutations are associated with the non-type I urinary amino acid pattern and the remaining 15% with type-I cystinuria.[34,36] The disease-causing mutations remain unidentified in approximately 15% of cystinuric patients.[32] These unexplained cystinuria cases may be the result of mutations in the promoter or intronic regions, the combined results of SLC3A1 or SLC7A9 polymorphisms in combination with specific cystinuria-causing mutations, or mutations in as yet unidentified genes.[32]

In dogs, cystinuria has primarily been diagnosed by analysis of the mineral composition of uroliths that have been removed from dogs suffering from some degree of urinary tract obstruction. Because of the availability of free urolith analysis at the Universities of Minnesota and California, a large amount of data has been accumulated. As for most types of uroliths, cystine uroliths are found predominantly in male dogs.[37–41] Approximately 1% of all uroliths in dogs in the United States are cystine stones,[39,40] with stone analysis laboratories in Europe reporting as high as 20% cystine stones (see, for example Refs.[42,43]). The mean age of dogs when cystine calculi are retrieved is between 4.8 years and 5.6 years.[37,39,43]

Urinary cystine crystals have a characteristic hexagonal shape, providing a useful diagnostic sign.[44] Cystinuric dogs can also be identified by analysis of urine for cystine. The cyanide nitroprusside reaction is a simple qualitative screening test for cystinuria, giving a positive result when 75-mg to 125-mg cystine/g creatinine are present in a urine sample. Quantification of all urinary amino acids by high-pressure liquid chromatography can also be performed but is expensive and not a routine veterinary test. In dogs, single urine specimens are collected without regard to time in relation to the most recent feeding. In contrast, in human patients, a 24-hour urine sample is analyzed, making correlations of the canine and human disease more difficult. However, when amino acid concentrations are adjusted to urinary creatinine concentrations,[26] there is a strong correlation between single sample and 24-hour cystine values.[45] Tsan and colleagues recognized the difficulty in diagnosing aminoaciduria from a single urine sample when he stated, "A low cystine value from a single urinary sample does not prove that the dog is not cystinuric".[46] There may be multiple factors contributing to this phenomenon, such as diet and diurnal variation in cystine secretion.[47]

Cystine uroliths have been recovered from dogs of approximately 70 breeds.[3,40] The following findings have been taken as evidence of a genetic basis: (1) increased incidence or risk of cystine urolith formation (based on data from urolith analysis laboratories); (2) multiple related cystinuric dogs or test matings that produce affected dogs; (3) detection of excess urinary cystine and dibasic amino acids or abnormal cystine renal clearance in urolith-forming dogs; and (4) urolith formation documented in female dogs. One or both of the first two criteria are found in several breeds (Australian cattle dog, Australian shepherd, Basenji, Basset hound, Bullmastiff, Chihuahua, Dachshund, English bulldog, Irish terrier, Mastiff, Newfoundland, Scottish deerhound, Scottish terrier, Staffordshire terrier, and Welsh corgi), while one of the four criteria has been observed in at least 23 dog breeds (reviewed in[48]).

Mating studies have been conducted for several breeds, beginning with the early studies of Irish terriers, where a cystinuric nephew of the propositus was identified[49] and additional matings produced 12 cystinuric dogs.[50] In a mating of a cystinuric male to two of his sisters, cystine urinary excretion was reported as slightly higher than normal in several dogs of one mating, while the other mating produced two cystinuric males and one cystinuric female. It was concluded that the inheritance of cystinuria was recessive, and while most affected dogs were males, an autosomal trait could not be excluded. The analysis of a Scottish terrier pedigree is suggestive of X-linked recessive inheritance.[46] In a similar study, only male Basset hounds were cystinuric.[51] However, all unaffected dams were siblings or daughters of cystinuric dogs; hence, autosomal recessive inheritance could not be excluded. Breeding studies in Newfoundland dogs excluded the X-linked recessive mode of inheritance and showed that cystinuria in this breed is inherited in an autosomal-recessive fashion. Aminoaciduria is present in male and female Newfoundland dogs at equal frequencies, with clinical signs predominating in males because of anatomic differences.[52]

Combined with breeding studies, urine amino acid analysis, and metabolic studies, cystinuria in Newfoundland dogs closely resembles the type-I disease in humans.[52] Affected male dogs formed cystine uroliths as early as 4 to 6 months of age, while females formed uroliths less commonly and later in life. Cloning and sequencing the canine SLC3A1 cDNA and genes from normal and affected animals revealed that affected dogs were homozygous for a nonsense mutation in exon 2 of the gene. This mutation results in a severely truncated protein of 197 amino acids, compared with the normal polypeptide length of 700 amino acids.[53] Testing for this mutation has been commercially available for several years, allowing breeders to detect which dogs are clinically normal carriers of the mutation and to choose mating pairs that cannot produce affected offspring. A similar mutation in SLC3A1 has been detected in cystinuric Labrador retrievers, which have a disease phenotype that resembles the Newfoundland type I cystinuria (P. Henthorn and colleagues, unpublished data, 2005).

While Newfoundlands and Labrador retrievers clearly have a severe (early age of urolith formation) type I form of cystinuria, the clinical and biochemical expression of cystinuria in other breeds seems to be quite variable. While some differences in various studies may be related to degree of clinical and laboratory investigation, as well as methodologic differences, multiple reports of variant aspects of phenotypes have emerged from independent sources over the years. These include variable cystine excretion in urolith-forming dogs, ranging from normal to approximately 100 times normal,[43] in both normal and elevated cystine excretion at different times in stone-forming dogs.[54] Variation in the underlying renal transport defect has been documented in renal clearance studies demonstrating variation from 50% of the normal reabsorption to active secretion within a breed and between breeds.[55] Multiple reports document urolith formation in dogs in which excess urine cystine concentrations were not detected.[45,56] These cases suggest that elevated urinary cystine concentration is not the only factor to consider as a cause of cystine urolith formation, as well as the possibility of a nongenetic form of cystinuria, where cystine urolith formation occurs in the absence of an amino acid transport defect.[43]

The estimated age of the dog at the time of urolith formation appears to be an important factor in classifying canine cystinuria. While the mean age at which cystine urolithiasis occurs in dogs is about 5 years, 11% of dogs form stones at less than 2 years of age,[57] with variation both between canine breeds and within individual cystinuric dogs of a breed.[43] Urolith-forming dogs with documented high urine cystine values that decreased with age to within the normal range[45] and apparent spontaneous resolution of cystinuria have also been observed in a Dachshund.[40]

Taking all the phenotypic and genetic data together, including breed-specific information, it is clear the canine cystinuria is genetically heterogeneous. Cystinuria in Newfoundlands (and also Labrador retrievers) clearly differs from the "average" phenotype of cystinuria in other dog breeds,[52] including higher incidence of urolith formation in female dogs and the juvenile age of urolith formation in male dogs.[40] In non-Newfoundland dogs, cystine and the dibasic amino acids appear to be excreted in the urine at lower concentrations than in Newfoundlands (**Table 2**). While the urine cystine and urine dibasic amino acid ranges in Newfoundland dogs[52] and those seen in 24 cystinuric dogs of other breeds[54] overlap, mean values for Newfoundland dogs

Table 2 Urine cystine and dibasic amino acid levels in normal and cystinuric dogs			
	Cystine	Ornithine	Lysine	Arginine
Dogs of nine breeds (not New foundland)[54] mean (SD; range)			
Cystinuric	368 (291; 17–1,115)	152 (215; 18–1,062)	1283 (1,558; 169–6,859)	177 (157; 12–655)
Normal	39 (26; 8–92)	39 (16; 9–73)	190 (58; 56–286)	84 (96; 14–335)
Newfoundland dogs[52] mean ± SD			
Cystinuric	1,081 ± 446	1,930 ± 2,414	3,494 ± 3,667	4,552 ± 5,173
Normal Relatives	54 ± 38	71± 36	143 ±102	83 ± 86
Normal Unrelated	<179	<202	<464	<452

While these values were not obtained from the same laboratory, examination of the normal values for each group indicates that they are roughly comparable.

are at least three times as high as for the group of the other 24 cystinuric dogs. There is also molecular evidence for genetic heterogeneity in canine cystinuria. Sequencing of the SLC3A1 and SLC7A9 protein-coding regions in a various breeds of cystine urolith-forming dogs of various breeds have not revealed disease-causing mutations.[53]

Based upon breed predilections, varied clinical features, and urinary amino acid patterns, there are at least two types of cystinuria in the dog. Type I cystinuria, documented in Newfoundlands and Labrador retrievers, is homologous to type I cystinuria in humans with mutations in the SLC3A1 gene. It is characterized by early age of cystine urolith formation in males, occasional urolith occurrence in females, and markedly high urinary excretion of cystine and the dibasic amino acids. Cystinuria in many other breeds is characterized by cystine urolith formation later in life (not before adulthood), moderately elevated and variable urinary excretion of cystine, and dibasic amino acids, with an as yet unknown mode of inheritance. Therefore, while mutations in one of the cystine transporter genes have been found to cause cystinuria in some dogs,[51,52] the genetic bases of cystinuria appear to be more complex than in humans. Discovery of the genetic basis of the more complex forms will undoubtedly rely on the new approaches made possible by the dog genome sequence.

ACKNOWLEDGMENTS

The authors thank Drs. Urs Giger, Margret L. Casal, Peter F. Jezyk , Kenneth Bovee, Stanton Segal, Junlong Liu, Angela Huff, Adam Sang, Tanya Gidalevitz, and Ping Wang for their contributions to the various canine cystinuria studies performed at the University of Pennsylvania. The authors also acknowledge the work of Drs. Noa Safra, R. Schaible, and G. V. Ling on hyperuricosuria.

REFERENCES

1. Smith BF, Stedman H, Rajpurohit Y, et al. Molecular basis of canine muscle type phosphofructokinase deficiency. J Biol Chem 1996;271:20070–4.
2. Ray J, Bouvet A, DeSanto C, et al. Cloning of the canine beta-glucuronidase cDNA, mutation identification in canine MPS VII, and retroviral vector-mediated correction of MPS VII cells. Genomics 1998;48:248–53.
3. Ling GV, Franti CE, Ruby AL, et al. Urolithiasis in dogs II: breed prevalence, and interrelations of breed, sex, age, and mineral composition. Am J Vet Res 1998;59:630–42.
4. Forterre S RJ, Kohn B, Brunnberg L, et al. Protein profiling of organic stone matrix and urine from dogs with urolithiasis. J Anim Physiol Anim Nutr (Berl). 2006;90:192–9.
5. Marangella M, Bagnis C, Bruno M, et al. Crystallization inhibitors in the pathophysiology and treatment of nephrolithiasis. Urol Int 2004;72(Suppl):1–6.
6. Carvalho M, Lulich JP, Osborne CA, et al. Defective urinary crystallization inhibition and urinary stone formation. Int Braz J Urol 2006;32:342–8.
7. Benedict SR. The Harvey Lectures. J Lab Clin Med 1916;1:346.
8. Moulin B, Vinay P, Duong N, et al. Net urate reabsorption in the Dalmatian coach hound with a note on automated measurement of urate in species with low plasma urate. Can J Physiol Pharmacol 1982;60:1499–504.
9. Wu XW, Muzny DM, Lee CC, et al. Two independent mutational events in the loss of urate oxidase during hominoid evolution. J Mol Evol 1992;34:78–84.
10. Alvares K, Widrow RJ, Abu-Jawdeh GM, et al. Rat urate oxidase produced by recombinant baculovirus expression: formation of peroxisome crystalloid core-like structures. PNAS 1992;89:4908.

11. Keeler CE. The inheritance of predisposition to renal calculi in the Dalmatian. J Am Vet Med Assoc 1940;96:507–10.
12. Safra N, Ling GV, Schaible RH, et al. Exclusion of urate oxidase as a candidate gene for hyperuricosuria in the Dalmatian dog using an interbreed backcross. J Hered 2005;96:750–4.
13. Roch-Ramel F, Peters G. Urinary excretion of uric acid in nonhuman mammalian species. In: Weiner KWIM, editor. Uric Acid. Berlin: Springer-Verlag; 1978. p. 211–55.
14. Roch-Ramel F, Wong NL, Dirks JH. Renal excretion of urate in mongrel and Dalmatian dogs: a micropuncture study. Am J Phys 1976;231:326–31.
15. Kuster G, Shorter R, Dawson B, et al. Uric acid metabolism in Dalmatians and other dogs. Role of the liver. Arch Intern Med 1972;129:492–6.
16. Giesecke D, Tiemeyer W. Defect of uric acid uptake in Dalmatian dog liver. Experientia 1984;40:1415.
17. Kocken JM, Borel Rinkes IH, Bijma AM, et al. Correction of an inborn error of metabolism by intraportal hepatocyte transplantation in a dog model. Transplantation 1996;62:358–64.
18. Vinay P, Gattereau A, Moulin B, et al. Normal urate transport into erythrocytes in familial renal hypouricemia and in the Dalmatian dog. Can Med Assoc J 1983;128:545–9.
19. Appleman R, Hallenbeck G, Shorter RG. Effect of reciprocal allogeneic renal transplantation between Dalmatian and non-dalmatian dogs on urinary excretion of uric acid. Proc Soc Exp Biol Med 1966;121:1094–7.
20. Schaible RH. Genetic predisposition to purine uroliths in Dalmatian dogs. Vet Clin North Am Small Anim Pract 1986;16:127–31.
21. Bannasch DL, Ling GV, Bea J, et al. Inheritance of urinary calculi in the Dalmatian. J Vet Intern Med 2004;18:483.
22. Albasan H, Lulich JP, Osborne CA, et al. Evaluation of the association between sex and risk of forming urate uroliths in Dalmatians. J Am Vet Med Assoc 2005;227:565.
23. Safra N, Schaible RS, Bannasch DL. Linkage analysis with an interbreed backcross maps Dalmatian hyperuricosuria to CFA03. Mamm Genome 2006;17:340–5.
24. Bannasch DL, et al. PLoS Genetics; in press.
25. Bende B, Nemeth T. High prevalence of urate urolithiosis in the Russian black terrier. Vet Rec 2004;155:239–40.
26. Treacher RJ. Urolithiasis in the dog—II biochemical aspects. J Small Anim Pract 1966;7:537–47.
27. Palacin M, Goodyer P, Nunes V, et al. Cystinuria. In: Scriver CR, Beaudet AL, Sly WS, editors, The metabolic and molecular bases of inherited disease, Vol III. New York: McGraw-Hill; 2001. p. 4909–32.
28. Lassaigne JL. Observation sur l'existence de l'oxide cystique dans un calcul vesical du chien, et essai analytique sur la composition elementaire de cette substance particuliere. Ann Chim Phys 1823;23:328–34 [in French].
29. Morris ML, Green DF, Dinkel JH, et al. Canine cystinuria. An unusual case of urinary calculi in the dog. N Amer Vet 1935;16:16–9.
30. Green DF, Morris ML, Cahill GF, et al. Canine cystinuria II. Analysis of cystine calculi and sulfur distribution in the urine. J Biol Chem 1936;114:91–4.
31. Calonge MJ, Gasparini P, Chillaron J, et al. Cystinuria caused by mutations in rBAT, a gene involved in the transport of cystine. Nat Genet 1994;6:420–5 [see comments].
32. Font-Llitjós M, Jimenez-Vidal M, Bisceglia L, et al. New insights into cystinuria: 40 new mutations, genotype-phenotype correlation, and digenic inheritance causing partial phenotype. J Med Genet 2005;42:58–68.

33. Palacin M, Estevez R, Bertran J, et al. Molecular biology of mammalian plasma membrane amino acid transporters. Physiol Rev 1998;78:969–1054.

34. Palacin M, Nunes V, Font-Llitjos M, et al. The genetics of heteromeric amino acid transporters. Physiology (Bethesda) 2005;20:112–24.

35. Schmidt C, Vester U, Wagner CA, et al. Significant contribution of genomic rearrangements in SLC3A1 and SLC7A9 to the etiology of cystinuria. Kidney Int 2003;64:1564–72.

36. Dello Strologo L, Pras E, Pontesilli C, et al. Comparison between SLC3A1 and SLC7A9 cystinuria patients and carriers: a need for a new classification. J Am Soc Nephrol 2002;13:2547–53.

37. Brown NO, Parks JL, Greene RW. Canine urolithiasis: retrospective analysis of 438 cases. J Am Vet Med Assoc 1977;170:414–8.

38. Case LC, Ling GV, Franti CE, et al. Cystine-containing urinary calculi in dogs: 102 cases (1981–1989). J Am Vet Med Assoc 1992;201:129–33.

39. Ling GV, Franti CE, Ruby AL, et al. Urolithiasis in dogs I: mineral prevalence and interrelations of mineral composition, age, and sex. Am J Vet Res 1998;59:624–42.

40. Osborne CA, Sanderson SL, Lulich JP, et al. Canine cystine urolithiasis. Cause, detection, treatment, and prevention. Vet Clin North Am Small Anim Pract 1999;29:193–211.

41. Weaver AD. Canine urolithiasis: incidence, chemical composition and outcome of 100 cases. J Small Anim Pract 1970;11:93–107.

42. Wallerstrom BI, Wagberg TI. Canine urolithiasis in Sweden and Norway—retrospective survey of prevalence and epidemiology. J Small Anim Pract 1992;33:534–9.

43. Hoppe A, Denneberg T, Cystinuria in the dog: clinical studies during 14 years of medical treatment, [erratum appears in J Vet Intern Med 2001 Nov-Dec;15(6):594]. J Vet Intern Med 2001;15:361–367.

44. Osborne CA, O'Brien TD, Ghobrial HK, et al. Crystalluria. Observations, interpretations, and misinterpretations. Vet Clin North Am Small Anim Pract 1986;16:45–65.

45. Hoppe A, Denneberg T, Jeppsson JO, et al. Canine cystinuria: an extended study on the effects of 2-mercaptopropionylglycine on cystine urolithiasis and urinary cystine excretion [see comment]. Br Vet J 1993;149:235–51.

46. Tsan MF, Jones TC, Thornton GW, et al. Canine cystinuria: its urinary amino acid pattern and genetic analysis. Am J Vet Res 1972;33:2455–61.

47. Lindell A, Denneberg T, Jeppsson JO, et al. Measurement of diurnal variations in urinary cystine saturation. Urol Res 1995;23:215–20.

48. Henthorn PS, Giger U. Cystinuria. In: Ostrander G, Lindblad-Toh, editors. The dog and its genome. Cold Spring Harbor(NY): Cold Spring Harbor Laboratory Press; 2006. p. 349–64.

49. Brand E, Cahill GF. Canine cystinuria. III. J Biol Chem 1936;114:xv–xvi.

50. Brand E, Cahill GF, Kassell B. Canine cystinuria V. Family history of two cystinuric Irish terriers and cystine determinations in dog urine. J Biol Chem 1940;133:431.

51. Albrecht F. [Symptoms, diagnosis, and treatment of cystinuria in the dog]. Kleintier-Praxis 1974;19:202–11 [in German].

52. Casal ML, Giger U, Bovee KC, et al. Inheritance of cystinuria and renal defect in Newfoundlands. J Am Vet Med Assoc 1995;207:1585–9.

53. Henthorn PS, Liu J, Gidalevich T, et al. Canine cystinuria: polymorphism in the canine SLC3A1 gene and identification of a nonsense mutation in cystinuric Newfoundland dogs. Hum Genet 2000;107:295–303.

54. Hoppe A, Denneberg T, Jeppsson JO, et al. Urinary excretion of amino acids in normal and cystinuric dogs. Br Vet J 1993;149:253–68 [see comment].

55. Bovee KC, Thier SO, Rea C, et al. Renal clearance of amino acids in canine cystinuria. Metab Clin Exp 1974;23:51–8.
56. Holtzapple PG, Rea C, Bovee K, et al. Characteristics of cystine and lysine transport in renal jejunal tissue from cystinuric dogs. Metab Clin Exp 1971;20:1016–22.
57. Wallerstrom BI, Wagberg TI, Lagergren CH. Cystine calculi in the dog—an epidemiologic retrospective study. J Small Anim Pract 1992;33:78–84.

Paradigm Changes in the Role of Nutrition for the Management of Canine and Feline Urolithiasis

Carl A. Osborne, DVM, PhD[a],*, Jody P. Lulich, DVM, PhD[a],
Dru Forrester, DVM, MS[b], Hasan Albasan, DVM, MS, PhD[a]

KEYWORDS

- Calculi • Uroliths • Nutrition • Struvite • Calcium oxalate
- Vesicourachal diverticulum

Results of experimental and clinical investigation have confirmed the importance of dietary modifications in medical protocols designed to promote dissolution and prevention of uroliths. The objectives of medical management of uroliths are to arrest further growth and to promote urolith dissolution by correcting or controlling underlying abnormalities. For therapy to be most effective, it must promote undersaturation of urine with lithogenic crystalloids by: (1) increasing the urine solubility of crystalloids, (2) increasing the volume of urine in which crystalloids are dissolved or suspended, and (3) reducing the quantities of lithogenic crystalloids in urine. For example, attempts to increase the solubility of crystalloids in urine often include dietary modifications designed to change pH to create a less favorable environment for crystallization. Increasing dietary moisture is commonly used to increase the volume of urine in which crystalloids are dissolved or suspended. Change in the composition of dietary ingredients is an example of a method to reduce the quantity of lithogenic crystalloids in urine.

This article summarizes and applies evidence about nutritional management of urolithiasis derived from experimental and clinical studies of cats and dogs performed at the Minnesota Urolith Center (MUC). How should this information be put into practice? For these studies to be of most benefit to patients, clinicians are encouraged to seek reproducible knowledge derived from properly designed clinical studies. Vigilance is necessary in order not to be misled by unsubstantiated anecdotes and dogmatic

---

This work sponsored in part by an educational grant from Hill's Pet Nutrition, Inc.
[a] Veterinary Clinical Sciences Department, Minnesota Urolith Center, College of Veterinary Medicine, University of Minnesota, 1352 Boyd Avenue, St. Paul, MN 55108, USA
[b] Hill's Pet Nutrition Inc., 400 SW 8th Avenue, Topeka, KS 66603, USA
* Corresponding author.
E-mail address: osbor002@umn.edu (C.A. Osborne).

Vet Clin Small Anim 39 (2008) 127–141
doi:10.1016/j.cvsm.2008.10.001
0195-5616/08/$ – see front matter © 2008 Elsevier Inc. All rights reserved.

myths. However, clinicians often have to adjust the application of scientific knowledge to meet the needs of individual patients. Frequently, there is no alternative but to extrapolate information derived from studies in one species for use in another. In this context, evidence-based medicine compliments rather than replaces the practice of compassionate medicine.

What is encompassed by use of the term "compassionate medicine"? The word "compassion" encompasses two different but complimentary components. First, we must have empathic awareness of the suffering, distress, or troubles of another. Second, we must have an empathic desire to help correct the problems.[1] Meaning well is not enough. Compassion moves us to come to the aid of those needing help. Thus, we must strive to attain and maintain our professional competence. This, in reality, is an extension of the Golden Rule (Do for others as we would like them to do for us). Stated in another way, we should strive to provide the quality of care that we would desire if we were the patients. Ethics demand that we not let ill-conceived treatment jeopardize the welfare of our patients. There are some patients that we cannot help. There are none we cannot harm. No patient should be worse for having seen the doctor.

FELINE LOWER TRACT UROLITHS
Epidemiology of Feline Uroliths and Urethral Plugs

Calcium oxalate was not the most common mineral in feline uroliths submitted to the MUC during the year 2007; of 11,174 feline uroliths evaluated, 41% (4553) were calcium oxalate and 49% (5432) were struvite. As has been the trend for the past two decades, struvite was the most common mineral detected in feline urethral plugs. Of 506 urethral plugs submitted to the MUC in 2007, 92% (463) primarily contained struvite and 1%[1] primarily contained calcium oxalate.

Calcium Oxalate

Medical protocols that promote dissolution of CaOx uroliths in cats are not yet available. Voiding urohydropulsion, lithotripsy, or surgery are currently the only practical alternatives for removal of active CaOx uroliths. However, clinical experience indicates that dietary management may minimize recurrence of uroliths or prevent further growth of uroliths remaining in the urinary tract.

Diet

The goals of dietary prevention include reducing supersaturation of urine with calcium oxalate, promoting higher concentrations and activity of inhibitors of calcium crystal growth and aggregation, reducing urine concentration and minimizing urine retention, and reducing exposure to nondietary risk factors. The complex interaction of various dietary ingredients on the formation and prevention of CaOx uroliths has been described elsewhere.[2] Provided patients are normocalcemic, epidemiologic and clinical studies indicate that recurrence of CaOx uroliths may be minimized by feeding a nonacidifying high-moisture diet formulated to avoid excessive protein, calcium, oxalate, and sodium.[2] The diet should contain adequate quantities of phosphorus so as to minimize renal activation of vitamin D, adequate quantities of magnesium, and vitamin B6. Avoid supplementation with vitamins C and D. Addition of citrate may be of value.

Outcome

Controlled studies designed to evaluate the efficacy of dietary modification in reducing the occurrence or recurrence of feline CaOx uroliths have not been reported. However, at the University of Minnesota, studies of cats with a history of CaOx uroliths revealed that the aforementioned dietary modifications significantly reduced the magnitude of supersaturation of their urine with calcium oxalate as measured by urine-activity product ratios.[3]

Sterile Struvite

Experimental and clinical studies have confirmed the effectiveness of a calculolytic diet in dissolving sterile struvite uroliths in cats.[4–7] In the authors opinion, dietary dissolution of sterile struvite urocystoliths is the preferred method of therapy for most cats.

Diet

Sterile struvite uroliths usually will dissolve in 2 to 4 weeks by feeding an acidifying high-moisture diet with reduced quantities of magnesium (Prescription Diet Feline s/d; Hill's Pet Nutrition, Topeka, KS). Because this feline struvitolytic diet is supplemented with sodium chloride, and because it is formulated to produce aciduria, neither sodium chloride nor urine acidifiers should be given concomitantly.

Outcome

In a clinical study of 22 (11 male and 11 female) cats, uroliths composed of sterile struvite dissolved in 20 cats in a mean of 36 days (range, 14–141 days) (**Figs. 1–3**).[5] Infection-induced uroliths require a much longer course of dietary and antimicrobic therapy. In one study, a mean of approximately 10 weeks was required.[5]

Prevention

Epidemiologic and clinical studies performed at the University of Minnesota indicate that acidification of urine and consumption of low-magnesium diets are effective in preventing recurrence of naturally occurring sterile struvite urocystoliths in male and female cats. No attempt was made to determine whether acidification or low-magnesium diets were the major factors responsible for beneficial results. The authors emphasize that reduction of some risk factors for formation of struvite crystals, including promoting formation of less alkaline or more acidic urine, is one of several risk factors for calcium oxalate urolithiasis.[2] Therefore, periodic evaluation of the patient to determine efficacy of dietary management is essential. If persistent calcium oxalate crystalluria occurs, appropriate adjustments in management should be made.

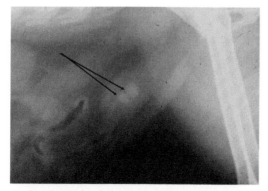

Fig. 1. Survey abdominal radograph of the lateral aspect of the abdomen of a 3-year-old spayed female domestic short-hair cat. There are two radiodense uroliths in the bladder lumen. Urinalysis revealed a pH of 7.5 and struvite crystalluria. There was no evidence of bacterial urinary tract infection.

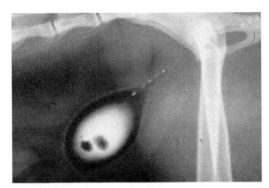

Fig. 2. Double contrast cystogram of the cat described in **Fig.1**. The uroystoliths appear radio-lucent compared with the radiodense contrast material injected into the bladder lumen.

CANINE LOWER TRACT UROLITHS
Epidemiology of Canine Uroliths

Of 28,629 canine uroliths submitted to the MUC in 2007, 41% (11,608) were struvite and 40% (11,577) were calcium oxalate. Purines comprised 6% (1737) of canine uroliths and cystine accounted for 1% (276).

Infection-Induced Struvite

Experimental and clinical studies have shown that infection-induced struvite uroliths in dogs may be dissolved with a litholytic diet and administration of antibiotics.[3,4,8]

Diet

The goal of dietary modification for dogs with infection-struvite uroliths is to increase urine volume and to reduce urine concentration of urea (the substrate of microbial urease), phosphorus, and magnesium.[8,9] The authors evaluated a high-moisture (canned) litholytic diet formulated to contain a reduced quantity of high-quality protein and reduced quantities of phosphorus and magnesium (Prescription Diet Canine s/d; Hill's Pet Nutrition, Topeka, KS). The diet was supplemented with sodium chloride to stimulate thirst and induce compensatory polyuria. In addition, reduction of urea from dietary protein reduces renal medullary urea concentration and further contributes to diuresis.

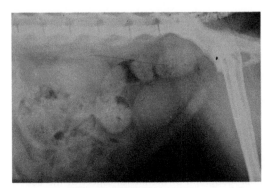

Fig. 3. Survey radiograph of the lateral aspect of the abdomen of the cat described in **Fig.1** obtained 4 weeks following initiation of dietary therapy to induce urolith dissolution. There are no radiodense uroliths in the urinary tract.

Antimicrobics

The importance of urinary tract infection with urease-producing bacteria in formation of most struvite uroliths in dogs emphasizes the importance of therapy to eliminate or control them. The authors used therapeutic dosages of antimicrobial agents selected on the basis of antibiotic dilution susceptibility tests. Preference was given to bacteriocidal drugs excreted in high concentration in urine, and with a wide margin of safety between therapeutic and toxic doses. The fact that diuresis reduced urine concentration of antimicrobial agents was considered when formulating antimicrobial dosages.[9]

Outcome

The efficacy of the aforementioned diet in inducing dissolution of infected struvite uroliths has been confirmed by controlled experimental and clinical studies.[10] The mean time for dissolution of naturally occurring infection induced urocystoliths was approximately 3 months (range, 2 weeks to 7 months) (**Figs. 4** and **5**).[8–10]

Prevention

Infection-induced struvite urolithiasis may be prevented by eradicating or controlling urinary tract infections.[9] For dogs with sterile struvite uroliths, Prescription Diet Canine c/d has been helpful.

Ammonium Urate

Clinical studies indicate that a litholytic diet and administration of allopurinol may be effective in dissolving and preventing ammonium urate uroliths.[9]

Diet

The goal of dietary modification for dogs with ammonium urate uroliths is to reduce urine concentration of uric acid. Because ammonium ion and hydrogen ion may precipitate urine uric acid, reducing urine acidity is also recommended. The authors used a high-moisture (canned) protein (purine)-restricted alkalinizing diet that did not contain supplemental sodium (Prescription Diet Canine u/d, Hill's Pet Nutrition, Topeka, KS). This calculolytic diet impaired urine-concentrating capacity by decreasing renal medullary urea concentration. The diet contained potassium citrate to promote alkaluria. When properly used, consumption of this food by healthy and urate urolith-forming dogs results in substantial reductions in urinary uric acid and ammonia excretion.

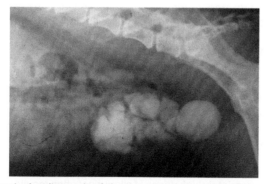

Fig. 4. Survey abdominal radiograph of the lateral aspect of the abdomen of a 12-year-old spayed female miniature Schnauzer. There are numerous radiodense uroliths in the bladder lumen. Urinalysis revealed a urinary tract infection with urease producing microbes, a pH of 7.5, and struvite crystalluria.

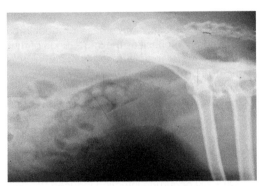

Fig. 5. Survey radiograph of the lateral aspect of the abdomen of the dog described in **Fig. 4** obtained 15 weeks following initiation of antimicrobial and dietary therapy to induce urolith dissolution. There are no radiodense uroliths in the urinary tract.

Alkalinization of urine

If urate crystalluria or hyperuricuria persisted despite appropriate dietary therapy, administration of alkalinizing agents, such as oral potassium citrate, was considered. Dosage of urine alkalinizers was individualized for each patient.

Allopurinol

Allopurinol decreases production of uric acid by inhibiting the conversion of hypoxanthine to xanthine, and xanthine to uric acid. The dosage that the authors have used for dissolution of ammonium urate uroliths in dogs is 15-mg/kg every 12 hours. Consumption of a high-purine diet while receiving allopurinol resulted in formation of a xanthine shell around urate uroliths or formation of xanthine uroliths. Therefore, allopurinol was administered only in conjunction with purine-restricted foods.

Outcome

At the University of Minnesota, 25 dogs with ammonium urate uroliths were treated with dietary and allopurinol therapy. Complete dissolution occurred in nine dogs (36%), partial dissolution occurred in eight dogs (32%), and no dissolution occurred in eight dogs (32%). The time required to induce dissolution of nine episodes of urate urolithiasis in this study ranged from 4 to 40 weeks (mean = 14.2 weeks). Inability to dissolve urate uroliths was often associated with formation of xanthine uroliths. In some dogs with partial dissolution, the remaining uroliths were completely retrieved using voiding urohydropropulsion.[9]

Prevention

Prophylactic therapy should be considered for dogs at high risk for recurrent urate uroliths. The risk for urate urolith formation may decline with age. As a first choice, diets that are restricted in purines and that promote formation of dilute alkaline urine should be considered. If urate crystalluria or hyperuricuria persists, alkalinizing agents may be added to the protocol. If difficulties persist, allopurinol (approximately 10 mg/kg to 20 mg/kg body weight per day) may be cautiously considered. Because prolonged administration of inappropriately high doses of allopurinol often results in formation of xanthine uroliths, it may be preferable to minimize the rate of urolith recurrence with dietary therapy, with the option of treating infrequently recurrent episodes of urate uroliths with dissolution protocols.

Cystine

Clinical studies confirm that a calculolytic diet and N- (2-mercaptopropionyl)-glycine (2-MPG) are often effective in dissolving and preventing cystine uroliths.[9]

Diet

Diets that promote formation of acidic concentrated urine are risk factors for cystine urolithiasis in susceptible dogs. These include high-protein dry diets, especially those rich in methionine (a precursor of cysteine). Reduction of dietary protein has the potential of minimizing formation of cystine uroliths. Pilot studies performed on cystinuric dogs at the University of Minnesota revealed a 20% to 25% reduction in 24-hour urine cystine excretion during consumption of a reduced-protein, sodium-restricted, urine-alkalinizing high-moisture (canned) calculolytic diet (Prescription Diet Canine u/d, Hill's Pet Nutrition, Topeka, KS) compared with a canned maintenance diet. An additional beneficial effect of protein-restricted diets was reduction in renal medullary urea concentration and associated reduction in urine concentration.

Urine alkalinizers

Oral administration of supplemental urine alkalinizers was considered if urine remained acid during dietary therapy.

Thiola

2-MPG (Mission Pharmacal) decreases urine concentration of cystine. Thiola was given at a dosage of 15 mg/kg to 20 mg/kg every 12 hours in conjunction with diet therapy to dissolve canine cystine uroliths.

Outcome

A combination of calculolytic diet and 2-MPG therapy was effective in promoting dissolution of uroliths.[9] With a combination of diet and drug therapy, the authors induced dissolution of 18 episodes of cystine urocystoliths affecting 14 dogs in an average of 78 days (range 11–211 days).

Prevention

Because cystine uroliths frequently recur in young to middle age stone-forming dogs within 12 months following removal, prophylactic therapy should be considered. Dietary therapy and, if necessary, urine alkalinization may be initiated to minimize cystine crystalluria. If necessary, 2-MPG may be added at a dosage of 15 mg/kg every 12 hours.

Calcium Oxalate

Medical protocols that will promote dissolution of CaOx uroliths in dogs are not yet available. Voiding urohydropropulsion, lithotripsy, or surgery are currently the only practical alternatives for removal of active CaOx uroliths. However, clinical experience indicates that dietary management may minimize recurrence of uroliths or prevent further growth of uroliths remaining in the urinary tract.[9]

Diet

The goals of dietary prevention include: (1) reducing supersaturation of urine with calcium oxalate; (2) promoting higher concentrations and activity of inhibitors of calcium crystal growth and aggregation; (3) reducing urine concentration and minimizing urinary excretion of calculogenic minerals; and (4) reducing exposure to nondietary risk factors. The complex interaction of various dietary ingredients on the formation and prevention of CaOx uroliths has been described elsewhere.[2,9,11,12] Epidemiologic and clinical studies indicate that recurrence of CaOx uroliths may be minimized by feeding a nonacidifying high-moisture diet formulated to avoid excessive calcium, oxalate, and protein. When selecting diets, a combination of low calcium and low oxalate content are preferred over other combinations. The diet should contain adequate quantities of phosphorus so as to minimize renal activation of vitamin D. Avoid supplementation with vitamins C and D. Addition of citrate may be of value.

Outcome diet

Controlled studies designed to evaluate the efficacy of dietary modification in reducing the occurrence or recurrence of canine CaOx uroliths have not been reported. However, at the University of Minnesota, studies of dogs with a history of CaOx uroliths revealed that the aforementioned dietary modifications (Prescription Diet Canine u/d Canned, Hill's Pet Nutrition, Topeka, KS) significantly reduced the magnitude of hypercalciuria and hyperoxaluria.[13]

Thiazide diuretics

Eight dogs with spontaneous CaOx urolithiasis received hydrochlorothiazide (HCTZ) (2 mg/kg every 12 hours) in a randomized, complete block (2-week treatment interval) design. Urine calcium concentration (8.6 ± 1.3 mg/dL to 3.7 ± 0.4 mg/dL) and excretion (1.6 ± 0.2 mg/kg to 0.9 ± 0.1 mg/kg every 24 hours) were significantly reduced and urine volume was significantly increased (20 ± 2 mL/kg to 26 ± 2 mL/kg every 24 hours) during HCTZ administration. Serum concentration of potassium remained within the normal range but significantly decreased (4.7 ± 0.1 mmol/L to 4.2 ± 0.1 mmol/L).[13] The hypocalciuric effect of HCTZ may help minimize recurrence of calcium oxalate urolith formation in dogs; however, long-term controlled clinical trials are needed to confirm safety and effectiveness of thiazide diuretics. Consider thiazide diuretics in dogs with highly recurrent disease; however, the authors do not consider thiazide diuretics as initial therapy because of the potential for hypokalemia. They may, however, be considered in dogs with highly recurrent disease.

ILLUSTRATIVE CASE REPORT
Recurrent Feline Hematuria, Dysuria and Pollakiuria: What Is Your Diagnosis, Prognosis and Therapeutic Plan?

The following case report illustrates several key concepts. The format is designed to request your viewpoints about diagnostic and therapeutic decisions. As questions are asked, please pause and think about your responses before continuing.

Database

A 3-year-old male, castrated domestic long-hair cat was referred to the University of Minnesota Veterinary Medical Center (VMC) because of recurrent hematuria, dysuria, and pollakiuria of 1 year's duration.

The clinical signs were treated with an antibiotic administered orally without long-term clinical response. The antibiotic was discontinued 1 month before admission to the VMC. The cat had been fed a dry adult maintenance diet ad libitum. Physical examination revealed that the cat was in good condition. Rectal temperature, pulse rate and rhythm, and respirations were normal. Palpation of the urinary tract revealed that the bladder was thickened and painful. Micturition induced by palpation resulted in voiding of a small quantity of bloody urine.

Analysis of a sample of urine collected by cystocentesis revealed that the urine was moderately concentrated (SG = 1.045), slightly acidic (pH by reagent strip = 6.5), and contained microscopic evidence of inflammation (pyuria, hematuria, and proteinuria). A few magnesium ammonium phosphate crystals of varying size were observed. Aerobic culture of an aliquot of urine revealed no growth. Results of a hemogram and serum chemistry profile revealed no abnormal findings. Re-evaluation of urine pH by meter was 6.8.

Problem List

What is your diagnosis?
Recall that the urinary tract responds to different causes (anomalies, infections, urolithiasis, neoplasia, and other potential causes) of disease in a limited number of ways. Classic signs of lower urinary tract disease are hematuria, dysuria, and pollakiuria. These signs localize the underlying problem to (at least) the lower urinary tract, but do indicate the cause.

Problems identified on the basis of the database include nonbacterial feline urinary tract disease characterized by hematuria, dysuria, and pollakiuria. The cause at this time is unknown.

Initial Diagnostic Plans

In your opinion, are further diagnostic tests justified at this time?
Because the lower urinary tract disease has been associated with these clinical signs intermittently for at least 1 year, and because the underlying cause is unknown, the answer is yes!

What is the likelihood of detecting the cause by radiography?
In terms of yield, the authors' experience is that survey abdominal radiography will reveal radiodense uroliths in approximately 10% of feline patients with lower urinary tract disease. Double contrast cystography will reveal uroliths in approximately 25% of patients with lower urinary tract disease. In contrast, quantitative aerobic culture of an appropriately collected urine sample from a 3-year-old neutered male cat can be predicted to yield positive results in about 1% to 3% of the patients. (Evaluation of unstained urine sediment is an insensitive method of detecting bacteriuria.) Therefore, with the goal of ruling-in (inclusion diagnosis) or ruling-out (exclusion diagnosis) urolithasis, radiographic evaluation of the urinary tract was recommended.

Follow-Up Studies

Radiographs of the abdomen revealed a solitary large radiodense urocystolith (**Fig. 6**).

In your judgment, is a contrast radiographic study of the lower urinary tract justified in this patient? What evidence can you cite to substantiate your recommendation?
Retrograde positive contrast urethrocystography revealed a vesico-urachal diverticulum at the vertex of the urinary bladder (**Fig. 7**). Additional uroliths were not detected.

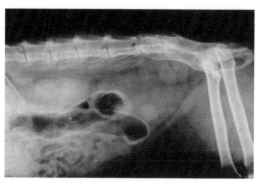

Fig. 6. Survey abdominal radiograph of a 3-year-old castrated male cat illustrating a radiodense urocystolith.

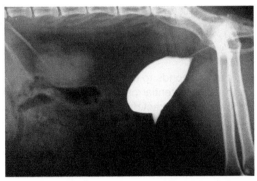

Fig. 7. Positive contrast urethrocystogram of the cat described in **Fig. 6.** Note the large vesicourachal diverticulum. The urolith has been obscured by the large quantity of radiopague contrast agent (Hypaque).

The cat was given a broad-spectrum antibiotic (amoxicillin and clavulenic acid) orally for 5 days following contrast radiography to minimize the possibility of urinary catheter-induced (ie, nosocomial) bacterial urinary tract infection.

On the basis of available data, can you predict the mineral composition of the urocystolith?

Would you choose ammonium urate, calcium oxalate, calcium phosphate, cystine, magnesium ammonium phosphate, silica, or some other type of mineral? What is the basis of your choice?

The authors' "guesstimate" of the mineral composition of the urocystolith was sterile magnesium ammonium phosphate (sterile struvite) because:

Bacteria were not identified by quantitative urine culture.

The urocystolith was large, radiodense, and had a smooth surface contour.

Magnesium ammonium phosphate crystals were the only crystal type observed in urine sediment. Ammonium urate, calcium oxalate, calcium phosphate, and cystine crystals were not observed.

The urolith was located in the urinary bladder (nephroliths are more likely to contain calcium salts).

The urine pH was only slightly acidic. In this range (approximately 6.5–6.9) of urine pH values, struvite crystals typically won't form but existing uroliths may grow.

How would you manage this patient if it were you, your family member, or your cat? Would you recommend surgical treatment, medical treatment, or a combination of the two?

In a prospective clinical trial of medical dissolution of feline magnesium ammonium phosphate urocystoliths performed at the MUC, consumption of a magnesium-restricted diet designed to promote formation of acid urine (Prescription Diet Feline s/d, Hill's Pet Nutrition, Topeka, KS) resulted in dissolution of struvite urocystoliths in a mean of 36 days.[5] Furthermore, the authors' studies have provided convincing evidence that most feline vesicourachal diverticula are a consequence rather that a cause of lower urinary tract disease.[4,14–16] Following elimination of predisposing causes (urocystoliths, infections, urethral obstructions, and so forth), most vesicourachal diverticula will heal in approximately 2 to 3 weeks.[15]

The client was given the option of surgery or medical therapy. The authors' discussed the benefits and risks associated with each procedure. Surgical removal of the urocystolith and vesicourachal diverticulum have the obvious advantage of rapid correction of these components of the disease process. However, surgery cannot be relied upon to remove subvisual uroliths or to prevent their recurrence. Likewise, surgery is associated with a higher risk of morbidity and mortality than medical management, although the risk of mortality associated with both types of therapy in this patient are low. The clients requested medical therapy consisting of a diet (Hill's Prescription Feline s/d diet-canned; Hill's Pet Nutrition, Topeka, KS) designed to dissolve struvite uroliths.

Considering the size of the urocystolith, what period of time would you predict will be required to dissolve the stone? When will the clinical signs resolve? When should re-evaluations of efficacy of therapy be scheduled? Will the vesicourachal diverticulum heal? If so, how long before healing is complete? Will vesicourachal diverticula recur?
Answers to these questions are provided in the following follow-up discussion.

Follow-Up Evaluation

When should follow-up evaluation be scheduled?
The authors have observed dissolution of struvite urocystoliths within 2 weeks of initiation of litholytic therapy.[5] In the authors' opinion, a follow-up evaluation of 2 weeks is optimum in that results of urinalysis provide insight into owner and patient compliance. However, a follow-up evaluation at 4 weeks is satisfactory, unless unexpected developments warrant more frequent observations.

The cat was re-evaluated 28 days after the initiation of therapy. The owner indicated that the clinical signs of hematuria, dysuria, and pollakiuria gradually subsided over a 2-week period following initiation of the litholytic diet therapy. Physical examination revealed no abnormalities.

Evaluation of a urine sample collected by cystocentesis revealed that the urine was concentrated (SG = 1.055) and acidic (reagent strip pH = 6.0). Crystalluria was not observed. The urine was yellow in color; however, a few red blood cells and white cells were detected by microscopic examination of urine sediment. The findings (acid urine pH, no struvite crystalluria) indicate owner and patient compliance with dietary recommendations. However, we did not achieve the goal of urine specific gravity <1.025.

Radiodense uroliths were not identified by survey abdominal radiography. Double-contrast cystoradiography revealed a small urocystolith (<0.1 mm) and marked reduction in the size of the vesicourachal diverticulum (**Fig. 8**). A positive-contrast cysotgram provided further evidence of urolith dissolution (**Fig. 9**).

The owners were shown before- and after-treatment radiographs to reinforce the need for continued therapy and to praise them for compliance with management recommendations. They were advised to continue feeding the calculolytic diet. They were also asked to give an oral broad-spectrum antibiotic (amoxicillin and clavulenic acid) known to be excreted in high concentration in urine for 5 days following double-contast cystography to minimize the possibility of urinary catheter-induced bacterial urinary tract infection.

The cat was re-evaluated 3 weeks later (7 weeks after initiation of therapy with the litholytic diet). During the 3-week interval between evaluations, the cat remained asymptomatic. Evaluation of a urine sample collected by cystocentesis revealed no abnormalities (SG = 1.052; pH = 6.0). Survey abdominal radiography, positive-contrast urethrocystography, and double-contrast cystography revealed no evidence of urocystoliths or the vesicourachal diverticulum (**Figs. 10–12**).

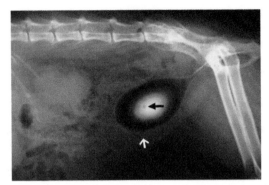

Fig. 8. Double contrast cystogram of the cat described in **Fig. 6** obtained 28 days following initiation of a litholytic diet designed to promote dissolution of struvie uroliths. Note the small urocystolith (*black arrow*) and substantial reduction in size of the vesicourachal diverticulum (*white arrow*).

What is the likelihood that the vesicourachal diverticulum might recur at a later date?
Based on current knowledge of the cause of macroscopic vesicourachal diverticula, the chance of recurrence is remote.[15] In the authors' experience with approximately 50 feline patients with vesicourachal diverticula, no recurrences of this structure after the co-morbid condition was eliminated or controlled have been encountered. Therefore, performing surgery to eliminate the likelihood of recurrence of vesicourachal diverticula is not based on sound evidence. In the authors' opinion, medical therapy should be the standard of practice in context of first-line therapy recommended to clients.

What is the likelihood of recurrence of urocystoliths?
Although there have been no controlled studies designed to evaluate the frequency of recurrence of uroliths, the authors' opinion, based 40 years of clinical experience, is that recurrence is an unpredictable event. Therefore, the owners were advised of the availability of diets designed to control the risk factors associated with the formation of struvite uroliths.

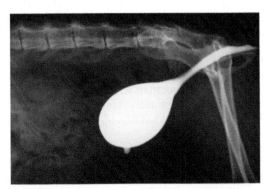

Fig. 9. Positive contrast urethrocystogram of the cat described in **Fig. 6** obtained 28 days following initiation of a litholytic diet. Note the reduction in size of the vesicourachal diverticulum described in **Fig. 7**.

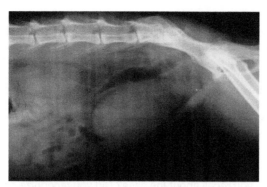

Fig. 10. Survey abdominal radiograph of the cat described in **Fig. 6** obtained 7 weeks after initiation of dietary therapy. There is no evidence of radiodense uroliths in the urinary tract.

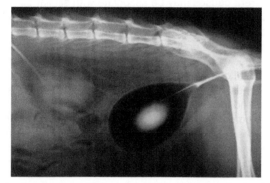

Fig. 11. Double contrast cystogram of the cat described in **Fig. 6** obtained 7 weeks following initiation of a litholytic diet. There is no evidence of radiodense urocystoliths.

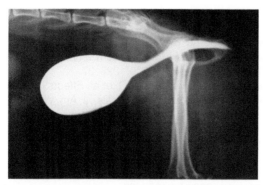

Fig. 12. Positive contrast urethrocystogram of the cat described in **Fig. 6** obtained 7 weeks following initiation of a litholytic diet. The vesicourachal diverticulum has healed. Compare with **Fig. 7**.

The need to periodically evaluate the effect of these diets on urine pH and crystal formation was emphasized, especially in context of the trend in the last decade of increased prevalence of calcium oxalate uroliths. While beneficial to patients with a history of sterile struvite uroliths, magnesium restriction and acidification of urine are considered to be risk factors for calcium oxalate urolith formation. The owners elected to feed a struvite urolith prevention diet. Periodic evaluation of the cat by physical examination, urinalysis, and survey abdominal radiography during the next 10 months revealed no evidence of lower urinary tract disease. Further evaluations were performed by the referring veterinarian.

SUMMARY

What key points do you recall about the case? Did you recognize any paradigm shifts in your thought process?
The points that this article emphasizes are:

The urinary tract responds to various diseases in a limited number of ways. A variety of different causes may be associate with similar clinical signs.

Survey abdominal radiography and double-contrast cystography are often be required to detect feline urocystoliths.

The mineral composition of uroliths may be predicted on the basis of knowledge of diet history, urinary pH, crystalluria, urine culture, radiographic characteristics of uroliths, and location of uroliths.

In the authors' series, struvite was identified as a major mineral in upper urinary tract (kidneys and ureters) uroliths in less than 5% of the samples.

Compliance with consumption of a magnesium-restricted diet designed to acidify urine typically results in sterile struvite urocystolith dissolution in a mean of 4 weeks (range, 2–6 weeks). Medical dissolution of feline infection-induced struvite uroliths with feline s/d and appropriate antimicrobics often requires a longer period.[13]

Vesicourachal diverticula often heal spontaneously within 2 to 3 weeks following eradication of the underlying comorbid disease.

The efficacy of diets designed to minimize risk factors for recurrent urolithiasis should be evaluated by periodic evaluation of the patient (especially urinalysis).

REFERENCES

1. Osborne CA. How can we become compassionate? J Am Vet Med Assoc 1992; 200:1082–4.
2. Lekcharoensuk C, Osborne CA, Lulich JP, et al. Association between dietary factors and calcium oxalate and magnesium ammonium phosphate urolithiasis in cats. J Am Vet Med Assoc 2001;219:1228–37.
3. Lulich JP, Osborne CA, Lekcharoensuk C, et al. Effects of diet on urine composition of cats with calcium oxalate urolithiasis. J Am Vet Med Assoc 2004;218:1583–6.
4. Osborne CA, Kroll RA, Lulich JP, et al. Medical management of vesicourachal diverticula in 15 cats with lower urinary tract disease. J Small Anim Pract 1989;30:608–12.
5. Osborne CA, Lulich JP, Kruger JM. Medical dissolution of feline urocystoliths. J Am Vet Med Assoc 1990;196:1053–63.
6. Osborne CA, Lulich JP, Kruger JM, editors. Disorders of the feline lower urinary tract. Vet Clin North Am 1996;26(Pt. 1):169–420.

7. Osborne CA, Lulich JP, Kruger JM, editors. Disorders of the feline lower urinary tract. Vet Clin North Am 1996;26(Pt. 2):423–665.
8. Abdulalhi SU, Osborne CA, Leininger JR, et al. Evaluation of a calculolytic diet in female dogs with induced struvite urolithiasis. Am J Vet Res 1984;45:1508–19.
9. Osborne CA, Lulich JP, Bartges JW, editors. The rocket science of canine urolithiasis. Vet Clin North Am 1999;29:1–306.
10. Osborne CA, Abdulalhi SU, Polzin DJ, et al. Current status of medical dissolution of canine and feline uroliths. Columbus (OH): Proceedings of the Kal Kan Symposium for Treatment of Small Animal Diseases; 1983. p. 53–79.
11. Lekcharoensuk C, Osborne CA, Lulich JP, et al. Associations between dietary factors in canned food and formation of calcium oxalate uroliths in dogs. Am J Vet Res 2002;63:163–9.
12. Lekcharoensuk C, Osborne CA, Lulich JP, et al. Associations between dry dietary factors and canine calcium oxalate uroliths. Am J Vet Res 2002;63:330–7.
13. Lulich JP, Osborne CA, Lekcharoensuk C, et al. Effects of hydrochlorothiazide and diet in dogs with calcium oxalate urolithiasis. J Am Vet Med Assoc 2001; 218:1583–6.
14. Osborne CA, Johnston GR, Kruger JM, et al. Etiopathogenesis and biologic behavior of feline vesicourachal diverticula. Don't just do something—stand there. Vet Clin North Am 1987;17:697–733.
15. Osborne CA, Kruger JM, Lulich JP, et al. Feline lower urinary tract diseases. In: Ettinger SJ, Feldman EC, editors. Textbook of internal medicine. 5th edition. Philadelphia: WB Saunders Co.; 2000. p. 1710–47.
16. Osborne CA, Kruger JM, Lulich JP, et al. Feline urologic syndrome, feline lower urinary tract disease, feline interstitial cystitis: what's in a name. J Am Vet Med Assoc 1999;214:1470–80.

Changing Paradigms in the Treatment of Uroliths by Lithotripsy

Jody P. Lulich, DVM, PhD[a],*, Larry G. Adams, DVM, PhD[b],
David Grant, DVM, MS[c], Hasan Albasan', DVM, MS, PhD[a],
Carl A. Osborne, DVM, PhD[a]

KEYWORDS

• Urolith • Urocystolith • Urethrolith • Nephrolith
• Lithotripsy • Calculi

In 1908, Drs. George Muller and Alexander Glass made the following statements about uroliths in dogs: "When the stone is present and causing retention of urine, there is nothing left but to remove the stones by means of an operation called urethrotomy if the stone is lodged in the urethra at the posterior end of the bones of the penis or cystotomy if the stone is located in the bladder."[1] One hundred years later, surgery remains a common procedure for rapid removal of uroliths from the lower urinary tract of dogs. Incorporation of intracorporeal laser lithotripsy and extracorporeal shock wave lithotripsy (ESWL) has provided impetus for a paradigm shift in the way veterinarians manage urinary stones, however. These minimally invasive techniques provide a successful alternative to surgical urolith extraction.

The term lithotripsy is derived from the Greek words "lith" meaning stone, and "tripsis" meaning to crush. A lithotriptor is a device for crushing or disintegrating uroliths. ESWL may be used to fragment and remove uroliths from the upper urinary tract, whereas intracorporeal laser lithotripsy may be used to fragment uroliths in the lower urinary tract by urethrocystoscopy.

INTRACORPOREAL LITHOTRIPSY

Successful medical application of intracorporeal lithotripsy depended on two technological advances: (1) delivery of energy capable of fragmenting uroliths without damaging adjacent tissue, and (2) cystoscopes capable of entering the narrow urethral

[a] Veterinary Clinical Sciences Department, Minnesota Urolith Center, College of Veterinary Medicine, University of Minnesota, 1352 Boyd Avenue, St. Paul, MN 55108, USA
[b] Department of Clinical Sciences, School of Veterinary Medicine, Purdue University, 625 Harrison Street, West Lafayette, IN 47907, USA
[c] Small Animal Clinical Sciences, Virginia Maryland Veterinary College, Virginia Tech, Phase II Duckpond Drive, Blacksburg, VA 24061, USA
* Corresponding author.
E-mail address: lulic001@umn.edu (J.P. Lulich).

0195-5616/08/$ – see front matter © 2008 Elsevier Inc. All rights reserved.

lumen to visualize and manipulate uroliths and their fragments. These technologies allow uroliths to be fragmented in the urinary bladder and urethra. Urolith fragments are retrieved with a stone basket or evacuated by voiding urohydropropulsion. Urolith removal is performed cystoscopically, obviating the need for a surgical incision.

Although several forms of energy (ultrasonic, ballistic, electrohydraulic, and laser) can fragment urinary stones, not all energy forms are suitable for use in companion animals. For example, the probes for ultrasonic lithotripsy are too large to pass through the operating channel of cystoscopes commonly used for dogs and cats. The ballistic lithotripter is too rigid to traverse the curvature of the male urethra. When treating humans, the safety and efficacy of electrohydraulic lithotripsy was inferior to holmium:YAG laser lithotripsy.[2] Because of the versatility and safety of laser lithotripsy, and the authors' familiarity with this treatment modality, the remaining discussion focuses on the use of holmium:YAG laser lithotripsy to manage urocystoliths and urethroliths in companion animal practice.

What Is the Origin of Intracorporeal Laser Lithotripsy?

The term "laser" is an acronym for Light Amplification by Stimulated Emission of Radiation. A laser is a device that transmits light of various frequencies into an extremely intense, small, and nearly nondivergent beam of monochromatic radiation with all the waves in phase. Lasers are capable of mobilizing immense heat and power when focused in close range.

Use of laser energy for intracorporeal lithotripsy is a relatively new concept. In 1968, investigators first reported in vitro fragmentation of uroliths with a ruby laser.[3] Because fragmentation of stones was associated with generation of sufficient heat that would likely damage adjacent tissues, however, it could not be used to treat patients. Likewise, use of carbon dioxide laser energy was considered unsuitable for clinical use because it could not be delivered through nontoxic fibers or through a liquid medium. In 1986 using a 504-nm pulsed dye laser, researchers successfully and safely treated human patients with ureteroliths.[4] The holmium:YAG laser is one of the newest and safest lasers available for clinical lithotripsy.[5,6]

What Is the Origin of the Name Holmium: YAG Laser Lithotripsy?

Holmium (Ho) is a rare earth element named after Sweden (the Greek word "holmia" means Sweden) in honor of the Swedish chemist who discovered it. A holmium:YAG laser is a laser whose active medium is a crystal of yttrium, aluminum, and garnet (YAG) doped with holmium (chromium and thulium), and whose beam falls in the near infrared portion of the electromagnetic spectrum (2100 nm). Several commercial models of holmium:YAG lasers for lithotripsy are available. The pulse duration ranges from 250 to 750 microseconds, the pulse energy ranges from 0.2 to 4.0 J/pulse, the frequency ranges from 5 to 45 Hz, and the power output ranges from 3.0 to 100 W. The power that one chooses is based on the desired application. The holmium:YAG laser that we use has a maximum power output of 20 W with a 350-microsecond pulse width (**Fig. 1**).

How Do Holmium: YAG Lithotriptors Fragment Uroliths?

The mechanism of stone fragmentation with the holmium:YAG laser is mainly photothermal, and involves a thermal drilling process rather than a shock-wave effect.[7] Laser energy is transmitted from the energized crystal to the urolith by way of a flexible quartz fiber. With each pulse, water at the tip of the laser fiber is vaporized creating a vapor bubble that when transmitted to the urolith causes thermal decomposition. Rapid expansion and collapse of vaporization bubbles shear the stone into fragments. To achieve optimum results, the fiber tip should be in direct contact with the surface of

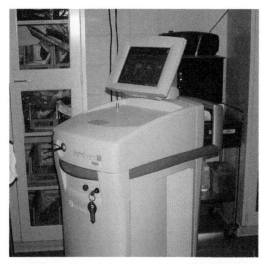

Fig. 1. The holmium: YAG laser (VersaPulse PowerSuite 20W Holmium Laser, Lumenis Inc., Santa Clara, CA) used to fragment lower urinary tract uroliths in companion animals.

the urolith during laser activation. If the tip of the laser fiber is not close to the stone (<0.5 to 1 mm), the surrounding fluid absorbs the energy and the stone remains unaltered.

Is Laser Lithotripsy Effective?

Laser lithotripsy has been reported to effectively eliminate urinary stones in humans, horses, goats and pigs.[5,8,9] In vitro studies revealed that the holmium:YAG laser consistently fragmented canine stones of all types (ie, calcium oxalate, cystine, struvite, silica, and urate) into extractable fragments (<3.5 mm in diameter) in less than 30 seconds.[10] These stones were immobilized during laser energy application in this in vitro study, whereas uroliths in clinical patients are freely mobile within the urinary tract resulting in longer lithotripsy times. Three studies designed to evaluate the efficacy of the holmium:YAG laser in dogs that had spontaneous uroliths report a complete urolith removal rate of approximately 82% to 84%.[11–13] In all three studies, complete urolith removal was achieved in 100% of dogs that had urethroliths (**Table 1**). In dogs that had urocystoliths, complete urolith removal rate was higher in females (83%–96%) than in males (68%–81%). In cases of incomplete urolith removal dogs were allowed to spontaneously void small (<3 mm) fragments, received medical therapy to dissolve uroliths composed of struvite, underwent successful voiding urohydropropulsion, had cystoscopic- or fluoroscopic-guided basket extraction of remaining fragments, underwent a successful repeat laser lithotripsy, or had residual stones removed by cystotomy. Reasons for terminating lithotripsy before complete urolith removal included (1) poor visibility because of urinary tract hemorrhage, (2) poor visibility or accessibility in males, (3) prolonged procedure or anesthetic time, and (4) lithotripsy-induced mucosal edema and perforation. Calcium oxalate was the most common urolith type in all three studies.[11–13]

Is Laser Lithotripsy Safe?

It is imperative to question whether lasers capable of fragmenting stones would also damage the adjacent tissues of the urinary bladder and urethra. Damage to the bladder wall is minimal, however, because the energy of the holmium:YAG laser is

Table 1
Advantages and indications for transurethral laser lithotripsy

	Rationale
Minimally invasive	Emphasizes the veterinarian's role to minimize unnecessary suffering
Rapid recovery	Compared to cystotomy, postprocedural urinary tract signs often resolve in 24 to 48 hours
Urethroliths	When held in position by urethral mucosa, urethroliths are often fragmented and cleared in minutes.
Urethral obstruction	Lasers quickly fragment uroliths restoring normal urine flow while obviating the need to perform disfiguring surgeries (eg, urethrotomy or urethrostomy) or retrograde urohydropropulsion. Success is high.
Pseudo-urolith recurrence	Unlike voiding urohydropropulsion, laser lithotripsy can safely manage uroliths immediately following incomplete surgical removal without a repeat surgery.

delivered in a pulsed fashion and readily absorbed by water. Continuous irrigation of the urinary bladder during lithotripsy therefore quickly absorbs and disperses stray energy. Under these conditions the thermal effect of the holmium laser is localized to within approximately 1 mm of the tip of the laser fiber. **Table 2** lists potential complications and strategies to minimize their development.

Bladder and urethral perforation, urethral swelling, hematuria, and leukocyturia have been reported in dogs whose uroliths were managed by laser lithotripsy.[11–13] In one patient iatrogenic perforation of the urinary tract resolved following transurethral catheterization for 3 to 7 days. Urethral obstruction due to urethral swelling also resolved following a few days of transurethral catheterization. In a similar manner, hematuria and inflammation abated by the third day following urolith removal. These results indicate that complications are short-lived and resolve spontaneously or with medical management.

When activated in room air, the force of the laser can travel approximately 1 m. Appropriate precautions should therefore be considered to prevent injury to those in the vicinity of an active laser. To prevent injury to people performing laser lithotripsy protective eyewear, safety shut-off devices, and operator training requirements should be reviewed before laser use.

How Is Laser Lithotripsy Performed?

Laser lithotripsy is performed by way of cystoscopy in anesthetized patients. Although patient positioning may be chosen according to operator preference, we usually place female dogs and cats in dorsal recumbency and male dogs in lateral recumbency (**Fig. 2**). Once uroliths are visualized with the aid of the cystoscope, the laser fiber is passed through the operating channel of the cystoscope (**Fig. 3**). The tip of the fiber is placed in direct contact and in a perpendicular orientation to the surface of the urolith. In our experience the initial energy setting to fragment stones should be approximately 0.6 to 0.8 J at 6 to 8 Hz. Energy settings can be increased as desired, but levels greater than 1 J and 12 Hz are rarely needed to efficiently fragment uroliths. During lithotripsy, sterile saline is continuously flushed through the working channel of the cystoscope to wash debris from the visual field and absorb stray laser energy.

Once uroliths have been sufficiently fragmented such that they are small enough to pass through the urethra, fragments can be removed by various methods. Initially, we

Table 2
Potential complications when performing transurethral laser lithotripsy

Complication	Occurrence	Avoidance
Bladder rupture	Rare	Bladder perforation is possible during excessive or forced overdistension with fluid, or from direct trauma by careless advancement of cystoscopes and laser fibers. Monitoring bladder fullness and cystoscope position minimizes iatrogenic trauma even in bladders with pre-existing weakness. Bladder perforation can also occur when incorporating voiding urohydropropulsion to remove urolith fragments. Keep the size and volume of urolith fragments to a minimum. Insuring adequate anesthesia to promote complete urethral relaxation minimizes excessive intravesical pressure during manual compression. If the integrity of the bladder wall is questionable, remove urolith fragments with a stone retrieval basket.
Cyanide production	Rare	Thermal decomposition of uric acid to cyanide can occur during lithotripsy. Our attempts to detect cyanide in the effluence during lithotripsy of uroliths composed of purines have been unsuccessful. Nonetheless, continuous irrigation of saline and frequent evacuation of the urinary bladder during lithotripsy is recommended to prevent cyanide from potentially accumulating to harmful concentrations.
Mucosal hemorrhage	Common	Hemorrhage obscures working visibility. In addition to strategies recommended to minimize urethral swelling, use lower laser power settings (0.6 J and 6 W) to minimize urolith ricocheting during urolith fragmentation
Mucosal perforation	Rare	Mucosal perforation is rare because holmium:YAG laser energy is delivered in 350-microsecond pulses and is quickly dispersed in fluid surrounding the tip of the laser fiber. Being careful that the laser is activated only when the fiber is in contact with the surface of the stone avoids urothelial perforation.
Retention of small urolith fragments	Common	Urolith fragments approximately 0.5 mm or less in diameter can become trapped in blood oozing from and attached to denuded urothelium. If not passed, fragments may serve as a nidus for future uroliths. Voiding urohydropropulsion 24 h or more following lithotripsy is often sufficient to completely evacuate the bladder. In some cases these minute fragments spontaneously pass during routine urine voiding
Urethral obstruction	Variable	Complete obstruction is rare because irregularly shaped fragments are unlikely to form an occlusive seal within the urethral lumen. Urethral obstruction may occur when large numbers of fragments are voided through the urethra simultaneously. If this occurs, use the laser to break up the fragment conglomeration and reduce fragment size. If anticipated, remove a portion of the fragments with a stone basket before voiding urohydropropulsion. Also see urethral swelling below.
Urethral swelling	Common	Urethral swelling impedes evacuation of uroliths and increases the likelihood of urethral obstruction. The degree of swelling is proportional to the frequency with which cystoscopes are passed and urolith fragments removed through the urethral lumen. To minimize this complication, pass well-lubricated scopes gently, select scopes with smaller working diameter than the urethra, fragment stones into smaller fragments before removal, and correct infection before lithotripsy. Also consider using a urethral access sheath to protect the urethra. If urethral obstruction is imminent, consider a short period (24 h) of continuous transurethral catheterization until swelling subsides.

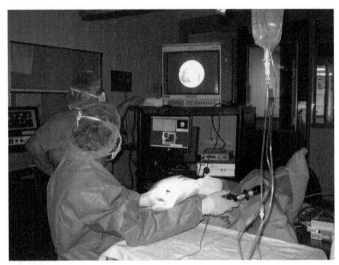

Fig. 2. Male dogs are placed in lateral recumbency to perform laser lithotripsy. The patient is placed under a sterile drape and a flexible cystoscope is inserted into the distal urethra.

use a stone basket to remove the largest urolith fragments. This procedure permits visual verification that urolith fragments have been reduced to sizes that will easily traverse the urethral lumen. Next, voiding urohydropropulsion is an efficient and rapid process to remove the remaining fragments. In most cases, however, we continue to remove the larger fragments by basket retrieval to ensure a successful urohydropropulsion at the end of the procedure. We adopted this approach to minimize the number of times a clean cystoscopy field needs to be re-established to retrieve retained uroliths with the stone basket or to repeat laser applications for fragments that fail to be expelled during voiding urohydropropulsion.

In some patients with substantial inflammation of the lower urinary tract, transurethral insertion of the cystoscope results in extravasation of blood and subsequent clot formation during lithotripsy. If the clot entraps stone fragments that remain adherent to the bladder wall, complete evacuation of stone fragments may not be possible. Our experience to date is that most of these fragments are less than 0.2 to 0.5 mm in diameter. Bleeding and formation of blood clots usually resolve in 24 to 48 hours. At that time, fragments retained in the bladder can be removed by voiding urohydropropulsion or can be allowed to pass during the voiding phase of micturition.

What Postlithotripsy Patient Care Is Advised?

Although cystoscopic evaluation of the urinary bladder and urethra with rigid endoscopes is sufficient for assessing urolith removal in female patients, the same degree of certainty is not achieved when using flexible fiberoptic endoscopes in males. Visual resolution of the fiberoptic scope is limited because the image is created from multiple individual fibers (**Fig. 4**). In addition, maneuverability within the bladder is limited because the fiberoptic scope only deflects in two directions and can only be rotated to a limited degree. For these reasons, we recommend a lateral survey radiograph and a lateral double-contrast cystogram to assess the lower urinary tract following lithotripsy. Inspection of the urethra with either type of cystoscope is sufficient to recognize residual urethroliths. Nonetheless, consider a positive contrast urethrogram in cases of considerable urethral trauma or suspected urethral perforation.

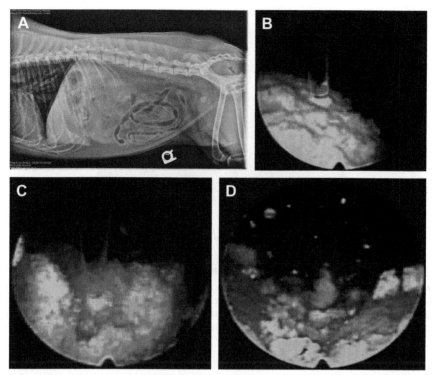

Fig. 3. Lateral survey abdominal radiograph of 4.5-year-old, 13.7-kg female dog that had a 1.2-cm urocystolith before laser lithotripsy (A). Cystoscopic view of the urocystolith undergoing laser lithotripsy (B); the laser fiber is placed in contact with the convex surface of the urolith to gradually fragment the urolith (C) into segments that could be easily removed through the urethra by voiding urohydropropulsion and basket retrieval (D). Laser lithotripsy was successfully completed in 56 minutes. The urolith was composed of magnesium ammonium phosphate.

We routinely provide antimicrobics (eg, penicillins, potentiated penicillin, or fluoroquinolones) for approximately 4 days to minimize iatrogenic development of urinary tract infection associated with insertion of the cystoscope through the urethra. Likewise, we administer medication to minimize urinary discomfort (eg, nonsteroidal anti-inflammatory agents or opioids); duration of therapy is variable (eg, 1 to 4 days) and based on the degree of urothelial trauma associated with uroliths and their removal, and continued based on duration of clinical signs referable to urinary tract pain.

Is Laser Lithotripsy More Effective than Surgical Cystotomy?

A case-controlled retrospective study compared 66 dogs whose uroliths were removed with laser lithotripsy to 66 dogs of similar stone burden whose uroliths were removed surgically.[14] Both were equally successful; for every eight procedures approximately one case required an additional procedure to complete urolith removal. On average, it took 23 minutes longer to manage urinary stones by lithotripsy compared with cystotomy. Patients undergoing lithotripsy were discharged from the hospital approximately 12 hours sooner. In another report of 23 dogs undergoing laser lithotripsy 84% were discharged the same day.[11]

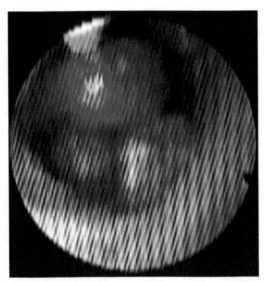

Fig. 4. Cystoscopic view of laser lithotripsy in a male dog using a flexible cystoscope. Image resolution with the flexible scope is lower because the image is obtained with a series of narrow optical fibers. The image resolution of the rigid cystoscope (**Fig. 3**B) is higher because the image is obtained though a series of rod lenses.

How Can Lithotripsy Procedure Time and Success Be Improved?

A common misconception is that patients can be maintained at a lighter plane of anesthesia during laser lithotripsy than during cystotomy or urethrotomy. This misconception is understandable because lithotripsy is a minimally invasive procedure in which tissues are not incised. Our experience, however, indicates that the level of anesthesia needed is equal to or greater than levels administered during traditional surgery. One approach that has been successful at maintaining sufficient anesthetic levels during lithotripsy has been the administration of a constant rate infusion of fentanyl (10–25 mcg/kg/h) in conjunction with inhalation anesthetics. A common complication associated with insufficient anesthesia has been hematuria attributable to the patient's urge to empty the urinary bladder during cystoscopy or constrict the urethra during voiding urohydropropulsion. In a few cases, hematuria was so pronounced and persistent that lithotripsy had to be postponed because of poor cystoscopic visibility. **Table 3** lists additional strategies to improve efficiency of urolith removal during laser lithotripsy.

What Factors Limit the Ability to Perform Laser Lithotripsy?

Urolith removal by laser lithotripsy may not be possible or ideal in all patients (**Table 4**). For example, cystoscopic evaluation of the urinary tract is not possible in male cats and some small male dogs because the urethra does not permit transurethral passage of a suitable cystoscope. In some cases urolith burden is excessively large such that surgical cystotomy is likely to be more efficient and cost effective. Although we believe that laser lithotripsy can be quickly learned, the cost of purchasing a holmium:YAG laser and cystoscopic equipment should be considered in terms of projected patient use. Additional accessories facilitating laser lithotripsy and urolith removal are provided in **Table 5**.

EXTRACORPOREAL LITHOTRIPSY

ESWL refers to fragmentation of uroliths using high-energy shock waves generated outside the body. The resultant small urolith fragments can pass spontaneously in the urine through the excretory pathway. On February 7, 1980, ESWL was first used to successfully fragment nephroliths in a human patient in Germany.[15] In 1984, the initial clinical trial of ESWL in the United States showed excellent fragmentation of nephroliths with extremely low morbidity.[16] Since that time, the widespread use of ESWL and subsequent development of intracorporeal laser lithotripsy have revolutionized treatment of nephroliths and ureteroliths in humans and resulted in a significant reduction in iatrogenic loss of renal function that was previously associated with surgical intervention for upper tract uroliths.[17,18] All common urolith compositions are amenable to fragmentation by shock wave lithotripsy (SWL) with the exception of cystine.[19] In humans, cystine uroliths have highly variable susceptibility to SWL with many cystine nephroliths being resistant to fragmentation.

A shock wave lithotriptor includes an energy source for generating the shock waves, a focusing device to concentrate the shock wave energy to a focal zone, a coupling medium to transmit the shock waves from the generator to the urolith within the patient's body, and an imaging system (fluoroscopy or ultrasonography) for positioning the urolith within the focal zone. Shock wave lithotriptors are referred to as water-bath or dry lithotriptors if the coupling medium used is a water bath or enclosed water cushion, respectively. The Dornier HM3 was the first-generation water-bath lithotriptor used in humans and is considered one of the most efficient lithotriptors.[20] Water-bath lithotriptors have been used to successfully treat nephroliths and ureteroliths in dogs.[21,22] Dry lithotriptors have also been successfully used to treat nephroliths and ureteroliths in dogs and ureteroliths in cats.[23,24]

How Is Shock Wave Lithotripsy Performed?

SWL is performed with dogs or cats under general anesthesia to facilitate positioning of the patient during the procedure and for analgesia. Application of shock waves during ESWL is painful and requires a depth of anesthesia comparable to abdominal surgery. For water-bath lithotriptors, the dog is positioned in dorsal recumbency at an oblique angle with the rear legs positioned lower than the front legs in a hydraulic gantry (**Fig. 5**). The gantry and patient are partially submerged in water such that the shock wave enters through the lumbar muscles overlying the kidney through the water. The front legs and head are not submerged under water to prevent risk for aspiration. For dry lithotriptors, the animal is placed in lateral recumbency and the enclosed water cushion is positioned against a shaved area of the skin overlying the urolith (**Fig. 6**). Careful coupling of the enclosed water cushion to the skin using generous amounts of ultrasound transmission gel is critical to permit passage of the shock waves from the shock wave generator into the patient. A potential source of treatment failure is poor coupling of the enclosed water cushion to the patient resulting in failure of transmission of shock waves into the patient.

The patient is positioned such that the urolith is within the treatment focal zone of the machine by targeting the urolith with fluoroscopy or ultrasonography. Lithotriptors vary in the size of the focal zone from 15 × 90 mm for the Dornier HM3 water-bath lithotriptor to 1.5 × 11 mm for Wolf Piezolith 2500 dry lithotriptor. In general, dry lithotriptors have smaller focal zones and require precise targeting for urolith fragmentation to occur. Furthermore, for lithotriptors with small focal zones, respiratory motion can move the urolith in and out of the focal zone.[17,20] Similarly, treatment of freely mobile

Table 3
Methods to improve effectiveness and efficiency

Strategy	Indication	Rationale	Procedure
Sufficiently deep anesthetic plane	When managing urethral stones, filling the urinary bladder with saline, or performing voiding urohydropropulsion, a sufficiently anesthetized patient will improve urolith removal	Sufficient anesthesia minimizes patient discomfort, mucosal hemorrhage, and inflammation.	In addition to providing adequate administration of a moderate level of inhalant anesthetics consider a constant rate of fentanyl (10–25 μg/h/kg) Administer propofol (1–2 mg/kg) as an intravenous bolus just before voiding urohydropropulsion.
Flushing urinary bladder before cystoscopy	Uroliths in male dogs	Reduced optical clarity of urine impedes visual inspection. The working channel of flexible cystoscopes is usually too narrow to rapidly empty and fill the bladder.	Using a large-bore transurethral catheter, empty the urinary bladder and rinse two to three times with saline. Following the final rinse, leave the bladder half full.
Use a V trough to position female patients	Uroliths in female dogs and female cats	V trough supports the patient during lithotripsy and voiding urohydropropulsion to remove urolith fragments from the bladder.	Position female dogs in dorsal recumbency. Instead of having to lift the dog up in the air, the trough near the head of the patient is tilted upward while keeping the opposite end of the trough stationary, allowing gravity to reposition urocystoliths for voiding urohydropropulsion.
Fluoroscopy	Uroliths in male dogs	The optical clarity and limited deflectability of flexible cystoscopes impedes lithotripsy. Fluoroscopy can improve operator orientation and urolith location.	Place dogs in lateral recumbency and center x-ray beam over the urinary bladder. With experience, we find that fluoroscopy is rarely needed.

Fragment bladder stones by first moving them into the urethra	Bladder stones in male dogs	Stone baskets and stone grabbers are used to retrieve stones from the urinary bladder and lodge them in the most distal portion of the urethra that could accommodate their size. Voiding urohydropropulsion can also be used to move bladder stones into the urethra.
	Sufficient hematuria to prevent visualization and safe laser fragmentation of bladder stones	Stones lodged in the urethra are held in place more firmly than stones in the urinary bladder. When the laser is activated they are less likely to be deflected out of the target zone. Because the volume of the urethra is small compared with the urinary bladder, blood can be efficiently cleared from the working area.
Occlude urethra proximal to stone	Urethroliths in male dogs	Proximal occlusion of the urethra prevents stones and stone fragments from returning to the urinary bladder where they are more difficult to retrieve and fragment. Insert a gloved index finger into the rectum and firmly occlude the lumen of the pelvic urethra by applying digital pressure against the ischium through the ventral wall of the rectum. Gently insert a lubricated catheter with a distensible balloon such that the inflatable balloon is proximal to urethral stones. Distending the balloon occludes the urethra.

Table 4
Relative limitations before considering transurethral laser lithotripsy

Limitation	Rationale
Bleeding disorders	Intravesicular hemorrhage obscures the operator's visibility to accurately aim the laser and retrieve urolith fragments
Small dogs	Although the urethra of most females can accommodate instruments to perform lithotripsy, the urethra of male dogs less than 6 kg may be too narrow for scope insertion or to safely manage uroliths by this technique.
Male cats	The urethra of the male cat is too narrow to accommodate passage of cystoscopes with working channels for laser fibers. Transurethral laser lithotripsy may be possible in male cats following perineal urethrostomy because the urethral lumen is wider.
Urethral stricture	Urethral strictures may impede the passage of cystoscopes and related equipment used to successfully perform transurethral laser lithotripsy.
Urinary tract infection	Urinary tract infection increases the propensity for urethral swelling and intravesicular hemorrhage during lithotripsy. Infusing the bladder with saline or manually compressing the bladder during voiding urohydropropulsion may reflux bacteria from the urinary bladder into the renal pelvises.
Excessive hematuria	Intravesicular hemorrhage obscures the operator's visibility to accurately aim the laser and retrieve urolith fragments
Large stone burden	Extended procedural time or additional lithotripsy procedures may be required to successfully fragment and remove all uroliths.
Small uroliths	Uroliths likely to pass through the urethral lumen should be managed by voiding urohydropropulsion or basket retrieval.
Equipment cost	Most veterinary centers purchased either the 20-W VersaPulse PowerSuite laser sold by Lumenis Inc. or the 30-W Odyssey 30 manufactured by Convergent Laser Technologies. Costs range from $40,000 to $60,000.

uroliths, such as cystoliths, may require repeated repositioning to effectively target and fragment uroliths, especially when using lithotriptors with small focal zones.

Once the urolith is positioned within the treatment focal zone, repeated shock waves are applied to the urolith and the urolith is monitored for fragmentation. Is it generally recommended to deliver a full therapeutic shock wave dose with each treatment to minimize the need for retreatment of uroliths.[20] For uroliths in the kidney and proximal ureter, the maximum number of shock waves should not exceed the safe limit for the lithotriptor used. For the Dornier HM3, the maximum number of shock waves that can be safely administered to the kidney of dogs without renal injury is approximately 1500 shocks. For uroliths in the distal ureter or urinary bladder, higher doses are possible because the kidney is not within the treatment focal zone and collateral damage to surrounding tissues seems to be minimal. One of the authors (LGA) has used up to 2500 shock waves during treatment of cystoliths and up to 4400 shock waves for treatment of distal ureteroliths without complications from these higher shock wave doses.

Is Shock Wave Lithotripsy Effective?

SWL has been successfully used to fragment nephroliths and ureteroliths in dogs and ureteroliths in cats.[21–24] In dogs, SWL treatment was successful in approximately 85% of dogs that had calcium-containing stones using the HM3 water bath lithotripter.[22] Overall approximately 30% of dogs required more than one SWL treatment for adequate fragmentation of their nephroliths. For dogs that have obstructed ureteroliths, approximately 50% required two or more treatments and some ureteroliths are not successfully fragmented with SWL. This finding is similar to research models that confirm that impacted ureteroliths are more difficult to fragment compared with nephroliths.[25] In cats, SWL successfully fragmented ureteroliths using large numbers of shock waves with dry lithotriptors, although success rates have not been reported.[24]

Is Shock Wave Lithotripsy Safe?

SWL is well tolerated by dogs that have normal kidney function. Likewise, SWL has a relatively low frequency of complications in dogs. In a series of 140 dogs that had nephroliths or ureteroliths treated by SWL by one of the authors, the most common complication was ureteral obstruction by fragments passing through the ureter, which occurred in approximately 10% of dogs treated by SWL. **Fig. 7** shows transient ureteroliths 24 hours after SWL fragmentation of large bilateral calcium oxalate nephroliths. Most of these dogs have transient self-limiting ureterolith fragments, but ureteral obstruction requiring intervention may occur during passage of fragments of nephroliths. Options for treatment of ureteroliths resulting from SWL include additional SWL to further fragment the urolith into smaller fragments, medical management to facilitate ureterolith passage, ureteral stent placement to bypass the ureteral obstruction, or surgical intervention (pyelolithotomy or ureterotomy). Other potential complications include shock wave–induced pancreatitis, which occurred in approximately 2% to 3% of dogs treated by SWL.[26]

What Patient Care Is Advised Following Shock Wave Lithotripsy?

Following SWL treatment, diuresis is recommended for 2 to 4 days to aid in passage of urolith fragments. Follow-up radiographs and ultrasonography are recommended 1 day following treatment and every 3 to 4 weeks thereafter. Urolith passage is rapid in some animals, whereas some animals may take several months to completely clear urolith fragments from the urinary tract. If the remaining fragments appear too large to safely pass through the ureter, a second treatment is recommended to achieve effective fragmentation.

Urolith fragments may be voided within 24 to 48 hours of SWL and voided fragments should be collected for quantitative mineral analysis to permit formulation of preventative strategies based on urolith composition. If urolith fragments collect in the urinary bladder and are not spontaneously voided within 1 to 2 months after SWL, then voiding urohydropropulsion is recommended to remove the urolith fragments.[8]

A PARADIGM SHIFT

The incorporation of laser lithotripsy and SWL has changed the way uroliths are managed in dogs and cats. With a 100% success rate in the management of urethroliths in dogs, laser lithotripsy abolishes the need to perform disfiguring urethrotomy and urethrostomy surgeries to correct urethral obstruction. Because these procedures are minimally invasive, most patients recover more rapidly without the need for restricted activity or devices or ointments to prevent premature suture or staple removal. Removal of urethroliths by lithotripsy allows us to put into practice the Golden Rule.

Table 5
Accessories facilitating laser lithotripsy and urolith retrieval

Accessory	Use	Additional Information	Source
Biopsy port sealers and adapters	Use to prevent backflow of fluid around laser fibers and other instruments being inserted through the working channel of cystoscopes.	Many types are available. Some are provided with devices such as stone retrieval baskets.	Check-Flow adapter (050,885), Cook Tuohy-Borst Adapter (TBA-6), Cook Urolok II Adapter (730-140), Boston Scientific
Ceramic scissors	Cut off the fractured and frayed end of the laser fiber before each use.	Laser fibers can be reconditioned and used repeatedly.	Ceramic Scissors (C-124) Kyocera Scribe Pen, Lumenis
Inspection scope	Use the inspection scope to evaluate laser fiber integrity before fiber sterilization and connection to the laser.	To prevent laser misfiring inspect laser fibers before each use.	Inspection Scope, Lumenis
Laser safety goggles	Protective eyewear is needed during laser operation	Laser lithotripsy is relatively safe. If the laser is accidentally fired when the tip is not contained within the urinary system, stray laser energy can damage the retina and other tissues in it firing path. Routine corrective lenses do not protect eyes from holmium:YAG laser energy.	Lumenis Numerous vendors
Laser ureteral catheter	Insert laser fiber into catheter so the tip of the fiber is not exposed. Insert both into the cystoscope. Before firing the laser, advance the end of the laser fiber out the other end of the protective catheter.	The catheter prevents the sharp end of the laser fiber from damaging the biopsy channel of flexible endoscopes. Catheters also minimize fraying the end of the laser fiber as it is passed through the biopsy channel of cystoscopes.	Laser Ureteral Catheter (022,402), Cook
Lithotripsy fibers	Flexible quartz laser fibers transmit laser energy to the surface of the stone.	Laser fibers are available in various diameters (eg, 200, 365, 550 μm) to accommodate the biopsy channel of any cystoscope. Energy delivered to fragment stones does not vary with fiber diameter; however, smaller fibers can be more expensive.	Laser Fibers (RBLF-200, 365), Laser Peripherals SlimLine 200, 365, and 550, Lumenis ScopeSafe holmium laser fibers, Optical Integrity

Device	Description	Comments	Product, Vendor
Narrow-diameter balloon catheters	In male dogs, use to prevent urethroliths and urethrolith fragments from migrating proximally out of the laser field. The balloon at the end of the catheter is positioned in the urethra proximal to the stone before its inflation.	Urethroliths are more efficiently fragmented because their movement out of the laser field is limited because of the minimal volume of the urethral lumen.	ClearView Silicon Foley Catheter, SurgiVet Many sizes and vendors
Single-action pumping system and tubing	Attach tubing to flush/biopsy port of flexible endoscope to facilitate administration of flushing solution.	The narrow flush/biopsy channel of flexible endoscopes minimizes adequate flow of flushing solutions. This device overcomes this impediment.	Single Action Pumping System, Boston Scientific
Stone grasping forceps	In male dogs, some stones can be retrieved and repositioned in the urethra to facilitate lithotripsy.	In general, stone grasping forceps permit easier stone disengagement than stone retrieval baskets.	
Stone retrieval basket	To reposition urocystoliths for fragmentation in the urethra and retrieve stone fragments following lithotripsy	Stone retrieval baskets are available in various sizes and types. Tipless baskets are preferred because they can retrieve smaller fragments. Many retrieval baskets are marketed for single use, but can be sterilized and reused.	NCircle Nitinol Tipless Stone Extractors, Cook Urological. Halo Nitinol Tipless Stone Basket, Sacred Heart Medical.
Stripper for laser fiber	Strip approximately 5 mm of plastic coating from the end of laser fibers before each use.	Laser fibers can be reconditioned and used repeatedly. A different gauge stripper is used for each different fiber diameter.	Microstrip precision stripper (Ms1-15s-18-FS), Slimline
Ureteral access sheath	A human ureteral access sheath is placed in the urethra of male dogs to facilitate clean and rapid access to the urinary bladder. A guide wire is used to facilitate placement of the access sheath.	Lithotripsy is often associated with repeated insertion and repositioning of the endoscope. The access sheath allows clean reinsertions without exteriorizing the penis of male dogs. The sheath protects the urethra from damage during instrumentation and stone retrieval.	Flexor (FUS-095,035), Cook
V Trough	V-shaped form padding facilitates positioning female patients in dorsal recumbency.	The trough also facilitates patient repositioning during voiding urohydropropulsion to evacuate stone fragments. Instead of lifting the patient, the trough is tilted such that the head is elevated to position stone fragments in the urethral outflow tract.	

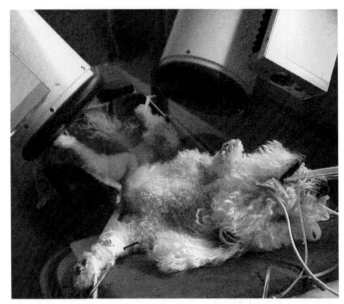

Fig. 5. An anesthetized female dog that had nephroliths is positioned in a water-bath shock wave lithotripter. The flash from the spark discharge that generates the shock wave is visible beneath the dog. Image intensifiers for biplanar fluoroscopy are visible above the dog.

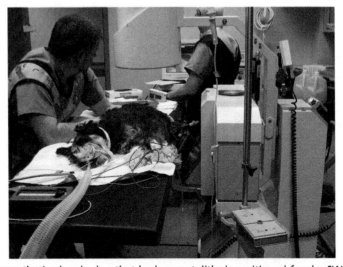

Fig. 6. An anesthetized male dog that had urocystoliths is positioned for dry SWL.

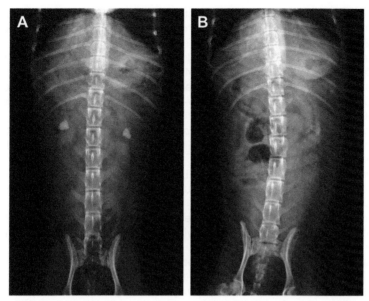

Fig. 7. Abdominal radiographs of a 9-year-old spayed female miniature poodle that had bilateral calcium oxalate nephroliths before (*A*) SWL and 24 hours after SWL (*B*) revealing multiple urolith fragments passing through both ureters. The fragments passed spontaneously without any associated clinical signs.

It brings us one step closer to completing our mission of making the surgical removal of uroliths a treatment of historical interest.

REFERENCES

1. Muller G, Glass A. Diseases of the dog and their treatment. 4th edition. Chicago: Alexander Eger; 1916. p. 199 (original copyright 1908).
2. Bagley DH. Expanding role of ureteroscopy and laser lithotripsy for treatment of proximal ureteral and intrarenal calculi. Curr Opin Urol 2002;12:277–80.
3. Mulvaney WP, Beck CW. The laser beam in urology. J Urol 1968;99:112–5.
4. Dretler SP, Watson G, Parrish JA, et al. Pulsed dye laser fragmentation of ureteral calculi: initial clinical experience. J Urol 1987;137:386–9.
5. Razvi HA, Denstedt JD, Chun SS, et al. Intracorporeal lithotripsy with the holmium: YAG laser. J Urol 1996;156:912–4.
6. Pierre S, Preminger GM. Holmium laser for stone management. World J Urol 2007;25:235–9.
7. Chan KF, Vassar GJ, Pfefer TJ, et al. Holmium:YAG Laser Lithotripsy: a dominant photothermal ablative mechanism with chemical decomposition of urinary calculi. Lasers Surg Med 1999;25:22–37.
8. Howard RD, Pleasant RS, May KA. Pulsed dye laser lithotripsy for treatment of urolithiasis in two geldings. J Am Vet Med Assoc 1998;212:1600–3.
9. Hallard SK, House JK, Geroge LW. Urethroscopic and laser lithotripsy for the diagnosis and treatment of obstructive urolithiasis in goats and pot-bellied pigs. J Am Vet Med Assoc 2002;220:1831–4.

10. Wynn VM, Davidson EB, Higbee RG, et al. In vitro effects of pulsed holmium laser energy on canine uroliths and porcine cadaveric urethra. Lasers Surg Med 2003; 33:243–6.

11. Grant DC, Were SR, Gevedon ML. Holmium:YAG Laser Lithotripsy for urolithiasis in dogs. J Vet Intern Med 2008;22:534–9.

12. Adams LG, Berent AC, Moore GE, et al. Use of laser lithotripsy for fragmentation of uroliths in dogs: 73 cases (2005–2006). J Am Vet Med Assoc 2008;232: 1680–7.

13. Lulich JP, Osborne CA, Albasan H, et al. Efficacy and safety of laser lithotripsy to manage urocystoliths and urethroliths in dogs: 100 consecutive cases. J Vet Intern Med 2008;22:732.

14. Bevan J, Lulich JP, Osborne CA, et al. Laser lithotripsy and cystotomy are equally effective for management of canine urocystoliths and urethroliths. J Vet Intern Med 2008;22:732.

15. Chaussy CG, Fuchs GJ. Current state and future developments of noninvasive treatment of human urinary stones with extracorporeal shock wave lithotripsy. J Urol 1989;141:782–9.

16. Lingeman JE, Newman D, Mertz JH, et al. Extracorporeal shock wave lithotripsy: the Methodist Hospital of Indiana experience. J Urol 1986;135:1134–7.

17. Lingeman JE, Lifshitz DA, Evan AP. Surgical management of urinary lithiasis. In: Walsh PC, editor. Campbell's urology. 8th edition. Philadelphia: WB Saunders; 2002. p. 3361–451.

18. Holman CDJ, Wisniewski ZS, Semmens JB, et al. Changing treatment for primary urolithiasis: impact on services and renal preservation in 16679 patients in western Australia. BJU Int 2002;90:7–15.

19. Williams JC Jr, Saw KC, Paterson RF, et al. Variability of renal stone fragility in shock wave lithotripsy. Urology 2003;61:1092–6.

20. Lingeman JE. Extracorporeal shock wave lithotripsy: development, instrumentation, and current status. Urol Clin North Am 1997;24:185–211.

21. Block G, Adams LG, Widmer WG, et al. Use of extracorporeal shock wave lithotripsy for treatment of spontaneous nephrolithiasis and ureterolithiasis in dogs. J Am Vet Med Assoc 1996;208:531–6.

22. Adams LG, Senior DF. Electrohydraulic and extracorporeal shock-wave lithotripsy. Vet Clin North Am Small Anim Pract 1999;29:293–302.

23. Lane IF. Lithotripsy: an update on urologic applications in small animals. Vet Clin North Am Small Anim Pract 2004;34:1011–25.

24. Lane IF, Labato MA, Adams LG. Lithotripsy. In: August JR, editor. Consultations in feline internal medicine. St. Louis: Elsevier Saunders; 2005. p. 407–14.

25. Paterson RF, Kim SC, Kuo RO, et al. Shock wave lithotripsy of stones implanted in the proximal ureter of the pig. J Urol 2004;171:294–5.

26. Daugherty MA, Adams LG, Baird DK, et al. Acute pancreatitis in two dogs associated with shock wave lithotripsy. J Vet Intern Med 2004;18:441 (abstract).

Canine Uroliths: Frequently Asked Questions and Their Answers

Lori A. Koehler, CVT[a],*, Carl A. Osborne, DVM, PhD[a],
Michelle T. Buettner[a], Jody P. Lulich, DVM, PhD[a],
Rosalie Behnke, MS, DVM[b]

KEYWORDS

• Urolith • Calculi • Question • Crystalluria • Urine pH

This article is devoted to answering frequently asked questions from veterinarians, veterinary technicians, and pet owners about urolithiasis. The authors do not stop with determining the mineral composition of uroliths; but also respond to questions related to the detection, treatment, and prevention of various types of uroliths from the urinary tract.

Originally it was suggested that this article be divided into veterinary and owner-related questions, but with the wealth of information available on the Internet, many owners have become quite curious and knowledgeable about uroliths affecting their pets, especially as it relates to nutrition. They frequently have many of the same questions asked by veterinarians and veterinary technicians.

The information has been divided into the following topics: urolith analysis, urolith types, diagnosis, treatment and prevention, urolith recurrence, urinalysis, diet, water, and miscellaneous.

UROLITH ANALYSIS
1. What Are Uroliths?

Answer: Uroliths are aggregates of crystalline and occasionally noncrystalline solid substances that form in one or more locations within the urinary tract. The urinary tract is designed to eliminate wastes in liquid form. When urine becomes oversaturated with lithogenic substances, uroliths may form and can interfere with the complete and frequent voiding of urine.

Supported in part by an educational gift from Hill's Pet Nutrition, Topeka, KS.
[a] Veterinary Clinical Sciences Department, Minnesota Urolith Center, College of Veterinary Medicine, University of Minnesota, 1352 Boyd Avenue, St. Paul, MN 55108, USA
[b] Hill's Pet Nutrition, 400 SW 8th Avenue, Topeka, KS 66603, USA
* Corresponding author.
E-mail address: koehl002@umn.edu (L.A. Koehler).

Uroliths typically are composed of one or more mineral types (**Table 1**).[1] These minerals may be pure, deposited in layers, or they may be mixed throughout the urolith. In addition some drugs may precipitate as crystals within the urinary tract and be incorporated into the urolith.

If foreign substances, such as suture material, hair, or plant material are present within the lumen of the urinary tract, they can become the nidus for urolith formation.

2. Why Should Uroliths Be Analyzed?

Answer: While guessing the mineral composition of uroliths by their appearance is sometimes possible, this method is subject to considerable error. Erroneous guesses of the mineral composition in turn often leads to formulation of erroneous therapy. Detection of the composition of the interior core of uroliths and/or microscopic surface crystals may also escape detection. To develop an effective treatment plan, knowledge of the composition and structure of the entire urolith is essential.

3. What Methods of Analysis Are Recommended?

Answer: Two general methods of urolith analysis are available: qualitative analysis and quantitative analysis.

Qualitative analysis is a colorimetric test designed to identify the chemical components of a substance or mixture. Drops of test reagents are added to an aliquot of pulverized urolith; the appearance of different colors indicates various anions or cations

Table 1
Crystalline substances that may be detected in uroliths

Chemical Name	Crystal Name	Formula
Oxalates		
Calcium oxalate monohydrate	Whewellite	$CaC_2O_4 \bullet H_2O$
Calcium oxalate dihydrate	Weddellite	$CaC_2O_4 \bullet 2H_2O$
Phosphates		
β-tricalcium phosphate (calcium orthophosphate)	Whitlockite	$\beta\text{-}Ca_3(PO_4)_2$
Carbonate apatite	Carbonate apatite	$Ca_{10}(PO_4 \bullet CO_3 \bullet OH)_6 (OH)_2$
Calcium hydrogen phosphate dihydrate	Brushite	$CaHPO_4 \bullet 2H_2O$
Calcium phosphate	Hydroxyapatite	$Ca_{10}(PO_4)_6 (OH)_2$
Magnesium ammonium phosphate hexahydrate	Struvite	$MgNH_4PO_4 \bullet 6 H_2O$
Magnesium hydrogen phosphate trihydrate	Newberyite	$MgHPO_4 \bullet 3H_2O$
Urice acid and urates		
Anhydrous uric acid	Same	$C_5H_4N_4O_3$
Uric acid dihydrate	Same	$C_5H_4N_4O_3 \bullet 2H_2O$
Ammonium acid urate	Same	$C_5H_3N_4O_3 \bullet NH_4$
Sodium acid urate monohydrate	Same	$C_5H_3N_4O_3Na \bullet H_2O$
Cystine	Same	$(SCH_2CHNH_2COOH)_2$
Amorphous silica	Same	SiO_2
Xanthine	Same	$C_5H_4N_4O_2$

that are present. Because this method requires pulverizing the sample into a sand of powdery consistency, the layers of different minerals frequently identified by quantitative methods of analysis typically cannot be identified by qualitative methods. Also, this method is not designed to determine the approximate percentages of different minerals that are present. Likewise, these tests are not designed to identify some biogenic components of uroliths such as silica or xanthine. In addition, crystalline drug metabolites are missed. One study comparing a qualitative chemical test to quantitative physical tests revealed false positive and false negative results. Test results were in agreement in only 92 of 223 cases.[2]

Quantitative methods of analysis are designed to determine the composition of a urolith, and the amounts or proportions of the components of a urolith. Several physical methods of quantitative urolith analysis may be used to determine and quantify the mineral composition of the sample. At the Minnesota Urolith Center, we most frequently use optical crystallography (polarized light microscopy) and infrared spectroscopy. On occasion, we use energy dispersive spectroscopy and x-ray diffraction techniques. Some laboratories include high-performance liquid chromatography to identify different forms of purines.[3]

4. What Is Optical Crystallography?

Answer: Optical crystallography encompasses the use of a polarizing light microscope to identify crystalline and/or noncrystalline components of uroliths by matching them to known refractive index oils. Representative sections of the urolith selected for microscopic examination are identified with the aid of a dissecting light stereomicroscope.

5. What Are Basic Principles of Infrared Spectroscopy?

Answer: Infrared spectroscopy is based on unique wave patterns generated when infrared waves encounter a sample. Some waves are absorbed by the sample (absorbance) and some waves pass through the sample (transmittance). The resulting spectrum is a molecular fingerprint of the sample. Because no two unique molecular structures produce the same infrared spectra, results can be compared with known reference spectra for identification. This procedure is useful in characterizing urolith components that cannot be identified with the polarizing light microscope, in determining the quality and consistency of samples, and for quantifying the amounts of different substances within the sample.

6. How Should the Results of Urolith Analysis Be Interpreted?

Answer: At the Minnesota Urolith Center, the following anatomic classification is used to describe different portions of the uroliths (**Fig. 1**).

Nidus—central area of obvious initiation of urolith growth, which is not necessarily the geometric center of the sample.
Stone—the major body of the urolith.
Shell—a complete, outer, concentric lamination of the urolith.
Surface crystals—an incomplete, outer lamination of the urolith.

Although all portions of the sample are analyzed, if all areas are composed of the same mineral composition, it is listed only under the "stone" area. Occasionally layers are encountered within the urolith or between the main layers that are listed as bands or incomplete bands on the report. Tiny focal deposits within the urolith may also be

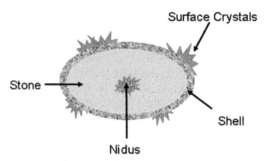

Fig. 1. Schematic cross section of a urolith illustrating separate areas that may be present. All layers are not present in all stones.

observed. These areas are included in the report if they are composed of a different composition then the other layers of the urolith.

7. Do I Need to Send All of the Uroliths Removed?

Answer: It is best to send a representative sample of all uroliths removed. Sometimes the larger urolith may contain a nidus layer that is not present in the smaller uroliths. Also, uroliths removed from different areas of the urinary tract may differ in composition. (See **Fig. 5** in "Changing Paradigms in the Frequency and Management of Compound Uroliths" elsewhere in this issue.)

8. If Only One Urolith Is Retrieved, Do I Need to Send the Entire Urolith for Analysis?

Answer: Submitting the entire urolith ensures that all layers of the urolith will be available for the most accurate analysis. Even if a sample visually appears to be homogenous, when examined microscopically, layers of different mineral composition may be present. (**Fig. 2**).

9. How Small Can the Sample Be to Be Suitable for Quantitative Analysis?

Answer: Because each lab is different, we recommend that you contact the laboratory providing the analysis to determine the minimum sample size. At the Minnesota Urolith Center, we generally indicate that if the urolith can be seen with the unaided eye (ie, the size of a poppy seed), we should be able to analyze it. Exceptions may include drug

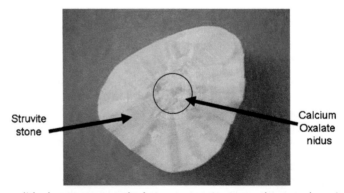

Fig. 2. The urolith above appears to be homogenous. However, the stone layer is composed of struvite and has a calcium oxalate nidus.

metabolites. Please note on the submission form alerting the lab of the small sample size (eg, Tiny sample enclosed).

10. What Should We Do If the Sample Has Been Fixed in Formalin Before Analysis?

Answer: Because formalin may alter or dissolve crystalline components, please send uroliths for mineral analysis dry. If a sample has been placed in formalin or other fixatives, and has not dissolved, remove the sample from the solution and allow it to dry. Please indicate that this sample has placed in formalin or another type of fixative on the urolith submission form.

11. The Patient Had Uroliths That Were Analyzed Previously. Should I Submit Uroliths Retrieved During the Most Recent Episode?

Answer: Yes. Recurrent uroliths may or may not be similar in composition to those retrieved in the initial episode. For example, development of a staphylococcal urinary tract infection in a dog that previously has a calcium oxalate urolith could lead to the formation of infection-induced struvite uroliths. In addition, dogs and cats are at risk for different mineral types at different stages of their lives. Therefore, we highly recommend that uroliths retrieved from each episode be analyzed.

UROLITH TYPES

Specific recommendations for each mineral type can be found at the Web site www. cvm.umn.edu, under *Departments and Centers*, then follow the prompts to find Minnesota Urolith Center.

12. What Is the Significance of Struvite and Calcium Phosphate in the Same Urolith?

Answer: Infection-induced uroliths also commonly contain small quantities of calcium phosphate. In most cases, therapy designed specifically for calcium phosphate is not required. In a few patients, the occurrence of calcium in struvite uroliths may be related to concomitant hypercalciuria. If therapy for struvite uroliths includes diets designed to promote acidic urine, the patient should be monitored closely for development of calcium oxalate crystalluria. Detection of persistent calcium oxalate crystalluria should prompt reevaluation of the strategy recommended for therapy.

13. What Is the Significance of Small Amounts of Ammonium Urate in Struvite Uroliths?

Answer: Infection-induced uroliths commonly contain small quantities of ammonium urate. In general, we recommend that therapeutic strategies designed to manage struvite uroliths be followed when considering management of these minerals. Therapy designed specifically for ammonium urate is not typically required.

14. What Microbes Are Commonly Associated with Formation of Struvite Uroliths?

Answer: Urease-producing *Staphylococcus intermedius* has most commonly been associated with the formation of canine struvite uroliths. Less frequently, urease producing *Proteus spp* and ureaplasmas (*Ureaplasma urolyticum*) have been associated with infection-induced struvite uroliths. Because *Escherichia coli* and other commonly isolated bacterial urinary tract pathogens do not produce urease, they are typically not a cause of infection-induced struvite uroliths.[4]

15. What Is the Value of Determining If a Urolith Is Composed of Calcium Oxalate Dihydrate or Calcium Oxalate Monohydrate?

Answer: Although different combinations of calcium oxalate salts have been identified in canine uroliths, the predominant form encountered has been calcium oxalate monohydrate (whewellite). Pure calcium oxalate monohydrate has been observed in dogs more frequently than pure calcium oxalate dihydrate (weddellite). A similar observation has been made in cats and people with calcium oxalate uroliths. When calcium oxalate salts occur in combination, the dihydrate salt is usually found surrounding a nucleus of the monohydrate salt.[5] The significance of this observation has not yet been confirmed, although it has been suggested that calcium oxalate dihydrate may form initially and then be converted to calcium oxalate monohydrate.[6–9] In humans, detection of calcium oxalate dihydrate on the outside of a urolith may indicate recent formation, whereas detection of external layers of calcium oxalate monohydrate indicates lack of recent urolith formation.[10] If valid in dogs, this hypothesis would be of clinical significance because it would help to determine if the disorders underlying calcium oxalate urolithiasis were persistent. This in turn would provide evidence of the need for continuous therapy to minimize urolith recurrence. In one study, human patients with calcium oxalate dihydrate uroliths had more recurrences of uroliths than did patients with calcium oxalate monohydrate uroliths.[6]

Calcium oxalate monohydrate and dihydrate uroliths are typically dense and brittle; they have relatively small quantities (~3%) of matrix. Pure calcium oxalate monohydrate and calcium oxalate dihydrate have different colors and shapes. In humans, uroliths composed of calcium oxalate monohydrate frequently assume the shape of mulberries or jackstones.[7] To date, only a few canine calcium oxalate jackstones have been observed at the Minnesota Urolith Center (**Fig. 3**). Calcium oxalate dihydrate most commonly forms rosette-shaped uroliths.

16. What Is the Frequency of Occurrence of Uroliths Other Than Purines in Dalmatian Dogs?

Answer: Between 1981 and 2002, the Minnesota Urolith Center received 9,541 uroliths from Dalmatian dogs. Of those uroliths 96% were composed of urates, 2%

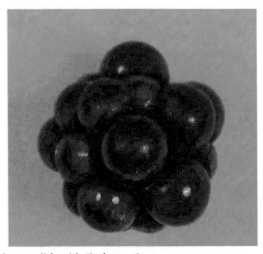

Fig. 3. Calcium oxalate urolith with "jackstone" appearance.

were of mixed composition, 2% were compound uroliths. Struvite, calcium oxalate, silica, cystine and calcium phosphate uroliths each made up less then 1% of the uroliths. Of these 9,541 samples: 93% were from male or castrated male dogs, 4% were from female or spayed female dogs, and 3% were gender unknown. Although urate uroliths are common in Dalmatians, other mineral types may also occur. Therefore, uroliths from all Dalmatians should be submitted for analysis.

17. What Is the Significance of Ammonium Urate Uroliths in Breeds Other Than Dalmatians?

Answer: The observation of uroliths composed predominantly of ammonium urate in non-Dalmatian dogs, should arouse suspicion that portal vascular anomalies or liver disease are the underlying problem. Provocative bile acids tests are recommended to rule in or rule out an underlying hepatic disorder. If liver disease is confirmed, dietary changes to reduce the urine concentration of uric acid and ammonium are recommended.

18. What Are the Similarities and Differences Between Xanthine Uroliths in Dogs and Cats?

Answer: Formation of xanthine uroliths can occur spontaneously or can be induced with the administration of the drug allopurinol. Acquired xanthine uroliths in dogs are usually an iatrogenic complication associated with treatment of urate uroliths with allopurinol. Similarly, xanthine uroliths can occur as a result of treatment of canine leishmaniasis with allopurinol. Naturally occurring xanthine uroliths have been found more commonly in cats than in dogs.[11] Cavalier King Charles Spaniels have been observed to have naturally occurring xanthine uroliths.[12]

19. What Are Some of the Contraindications of Allopurinol Therapy?

Answer: The use of allopurinol therapy in dogs can lead to the iatrogenic formation of xanthine crystalluria and uroliths. Unfortunately xanthine and urate crystals cannot be easily differentiated from each other by polarizing microscopy. If large quantities of crystals are present in the urine, infrared spectroscopy can be performed to differentiate the crystal type. In a study of healthy beagles, urinary excretion of xanthine was measured in dogs fed a low-protein, casein-based diet versus a high-protein, meat-based diet. When consuming the high-protein diet and allopurinol, urinary xanthine excretion was significantly higher. Therefore, if dietary compliance with a low-protein diet is not followed, and treats or an inappropriately high purine diet is fed, the possibility of xanthine formation increases.[13]

20. What Are the Similarities and Differences Between Cystine Uroliths in Dogs and Cats?

Answer: Cystinuria is an inborn error of metabolism causing impaired renal tubular reabsorption of the relatively insoluble nonessential dibasic sulfur containing amino acid cystine. Renal excretion of other dibasic amino acids may also be altered. Cystinuria predisposes affected dogs and cats to formation of highly recurrent cystine uroliths. Dietary management and drug therapy have been used to dissolve cystine uroliths in dogs. However, studies to determine the safety and efficacy of drug therapy in cats is still pending. Canine cystine uroliths are encountered most commonly in males.[14] The Minnesota Urolith Center analyzed 1,928 canine cystine uroliths submitted between 2000 and 2006. Over 90 breeds were affected; the breeds most commonly affected were: English Bulldogs (18%), mixed breed dogs (6%), Dachshunds (6%), Staffordshire Bull Terriers (6%), Mastiffs (6%), and Chihuahuas (5%).

21. What About Prevention of Uroliths Composed of Two Different Mineral Types that Have Opposite Risk Factors?

Answer: A variety of mineral combinations can occur in compound uroliths. For information related to dissolution and prevention, please see the article entitled, "Changing Paradigms in the Frequency and Management of Compound Uroliths" elsewhere in this issue.

22. The Urolith Results Indicated that a Hollow Cylindrical Central Area Was Present. Why Did This Hollow Area Form?

Answer: Please refer to the article entitled, "Changing Paradigms in the Frequency and Management of Compound Uroilths" elsewhere in this issue for information about this phenomenon.

23. What About Foreign Material (Bodies) Found Inside the Urolith?

Answer: Please refer to the article entitled, "Changing Paradigms in the Frequency and Management of Compound Uroliths" elsewhere in this issue for details about foreign objects found in uroliths.

24. Is Calcium Carbonate a Common Primary Mineral Type in Dogs?

Answer: No. At the Minnesota Urolith Center we have only found 6 of 350,803 canine uroliths submitted from 1981 to 2007 to be composed primarily of calcium carbonate. We occasionally find calcium carbonate as a minor component of canine and feline uroliths, but are unsure of its significance. In contrast, calcium carbonate is a common primary mineral type in horses, rabbits, guinea pigs, and goats.

25. What About Stones Formed in Other Locations, Such As Cholecystoliths, Pancreatoliths, and Sialoliths?

Answer: Stones do occur in these locations in animals. In most cases, the mineral composition of these stones can be analyzed by the same quantitative techniques used to analyze urocystoliths. Please contact the Minnesota Urolith Center if you have specific questions.

DIAGNOSIS
26. Do Uroliths Have a Characteristic Appearance?

Answer: Most uroliths have typical appearances or "habits." For example, struvite uroliths often are light tan and have a pyramidal or oval shape. Another noticeable example is silica uroliths having a jackstone appearance. However, we commonly receive samples that do not have the typical appearance characteristics. (**Figs. 4** and **5**).

In addition, the inner composition of a urolith cannot reliably be predicted by evaluating the appearance of its outer surface. In our series of canine uroliths analyzed from 1981 to 2007, 9% of uroliths were classified as compound.

27. How can the Mineral Composition of Uroliths be Determined if All of the Uroliths are Still in the Patient?

Answer: Urolith composition can often be "guesstimated" by looking at relevant clinical findings including results of radiography, urinalysis, urine culture and the patients breed, age, and gender (see **Table 2**). For additional information about interpreting radiographic findings, the article "Changing Paradigms in the Frequency and Management of Compound Uroliths" elsewhere in this issue.

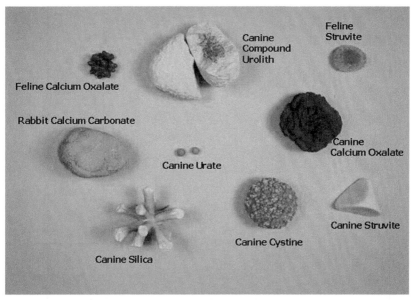

Fig. 4. Characteristic shapes of various urolith types.

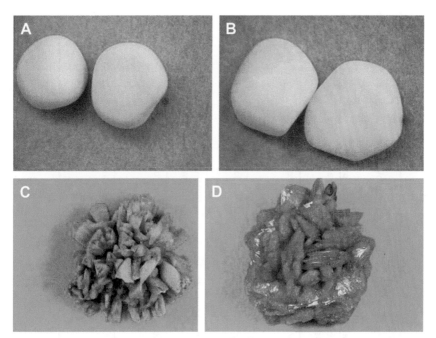

Fig. 5. Photos above demonstrate how uroliths of different composition can have similar appearances. (*A*) Cystine. (*B*) Magnesium ammonium phosphate. (*C*) Magnesium ammonium phosphate. (*D*) Calcium oxalate.

Table 2
Checklist of factors that suggest the probable mineral composition of canine uroliths

Mineral Type	Urine pH	Radiographic Density	Breed Predisposition	Gender Predisposition	Common Age (y)
Magnesium ammonium phosphate	Neutral to alkaline	+ to ++++	Miniature Schnauzer, Shih Tzu, Yorkshire Terrier, Pug, Labrador, Dachshund	Female (>85%)	2–9
Calcium oxalate	Acid to neutral	++ to ++++	Bichon Frise, Lhasa Apso, Miniature Schnauzer, Pomeranian, Shih Tzu, Yorkshire Terrier	Male (>70%)	5–11
Purine, including urate	Acid to neutral	0 to ++	Dalmatian, English Bulldog, Miniature Schnauzer, Shih Tzu, Yorkshire Terrier	Male (>85%)	1–4
Calcium phosphate	Alkaline to neutral (brushite forms in acid urine)	++ to ++++	Bichon Frise, Miniature Poodle, Pomeranian, Pug, Shih Tzu, Yorkshire Terrier	Male (>53%)	<1; 6–10
Cystine	Acid to neutral	+ to ++	English Bulldog, Staffordshire Bull Terrier, Mastiff, Dachshund, Chihuahua, Newfoundland	Males (>94%)	1–7
Silica	Acid to neutral	++ to +++	German Shepherd, Labrador, Shih Tzu, Yorkshire Terrier, Rottweiler, Boxer, Bichon Frise	Male (>92%)	3–10

28. How Is it Possible for the Patient to Have Uroliths Without Crystalluria?

Answer: The absence of crystalluria in patients with confirmed uroliths indicates that at the time urine was collected, it was not oversaturated with substances required for the formation of crystals. Detection of crystalluria is not synonymous with the presence of uroliths.[15] However, the fact that crystals were not observed is often a positive observation because it should be possible to induce the same environment and at least minimize further stone growth. For further information, refer to question 48 about one cause of in vitro crystalluria.

29. A Neutered Male Schnauzer Has Bladder Stones. Can I Dissolve Them?

Answer: Refer to **Table 2**. Consideration of the dog's age, urinalysis or culture results, and radiographic findings will help guesstimate what type of urolith the patient has and if it can be dissolved. Miniature Schnauzers are at risk for forming a variety of different urolith types. Miniature Schnauzers comprised 9% of struvite uroliths, 4% of urate uroliths, and 18% of calcium oxalate uroliths submitted to the Minnesota Urolith Center between 2000 and 2006.

TREATMENT AND PREVENTION
30. What Are the Most Important Steps to Consider when Minimizing Recurrence of Uroliths?

Answer

- Be certain that you have an accurate diagnosis.
- Correct any underlying conditions, such as urinary tract infections or hypercalcemia.
- Promote less concentrated urine, aiming for a specific gravity <1.020.
- Monitor the patient at appropriate intervals to identify potential recurrences early.

31. How Important Is the Recommendation to Periodically Monitor the Patient for Recurrence?

Answer: All prevention recommendations should be periodically monitored and adjusted to meet each individual patient's needs. This typically includes follow-up urinalyses, serum chemistry profiles, and radiography. Early detection of small urocystoliths that recur despite appropriate medical therapy facilitates nonsurgical removal by voiding urohydropropulsion.[16]

See question 42 for information about recurrence rates of different mineral types.

32. How Do I Decide to Try Dissolution Versus Other Methods of Urolith Removal?

Answer: If the uroliths are small enough, voiding or catheter retrieval may be possible. The advantage of these techniques is that retrieved uroliths can then be analyzed to determine appropriate dissolution or prevention protocols. Before attempting dissolution, perform diagnostic studies (urinalysis, urine culture, radiography, analysis of voided uroliths, etc.) to evaluate urolith size and location, as well as confirmation of urolith composition. Urethroliths and ureteroliths cannot be dissolved by medical protocols (See question 34). Discuss the cost of diet and antibiotic therapy with the owner. Also inform them of the estimated cost and the desirability of recheck appointments, when providing them with the option of medical dissolution. Some owners avoid surgical procedures for their pets and will elect to try the option of dissolution first. Other clients may feel that their pet is uncomfortable and will elect to have the uroliths surgically removed. When formulating medical dissolution protocols, be sure to discuss the need for compliance with your recommendations with the owner.

If a reduction in urolith size or numbers is not seen by medical imaging techniques after 4 to 6 weeks, reassess the patient and consider other options. Regardless of the management selected, the owner should be advised of the need for periodic monitoring. See question 31.

33. What Sizes or Number of Uroliths Makes the Candidate a Poor Candidate for Medical Dissolution?

Answer: The size and number of uroliths do not dictate the likelihood of response to therapy. We have had success in dissolving uroliths that are small and large, single and multiple. However, the rate of dissolution is related to size and surface area of the urolith exposed to urine. Just as one large ice cube dissolves in water more slowly than an equal volume of crushed ice, one large urolith will dissolve more slowly in urine than an equal volume of many smaller uroliths. The rate of dissolution is influenced by surface area of the urolith exposed to undersaturated urine.[16]

34. Can Struvite Uroliths Located in the Urethra or Ureters Be Dissolved Medically?

Answer: Urolith dissolution requires sustained contact of uroliths with urine that has been modified so that it is undersaturated with lithogenic minerals. Struvite, urate, or cystine uroliths located in the ureters or urethra cannot be dissolved by medical protocols because they are only intermittently in contact with urine. If urethroliths are returned to the urinary bladder by retrograde urohydropulsion, they may be subsequently managed by medical dissolution, lithotripsy, or surgery.[16]

35. The Patient Voided a Few Small Uroliths that Were Composed of Struvite, with a Shell of Calcium Phosphate Carbonate. What Is the Likelihood that Uroliths of Similar Composition Remaining in the Bladder Can Be Dissolved?

Answer: Please refer to the article entitled, "Changing Paradigms in Compound Uroliths" in this edition of Veterinary Clinics of North America for specific information about compound uroliths.

36. The Nidus and Stone Layers of the Urolith Have Very Different Mineral Components. Recommendations to Dissolve the Uroliths and to Minimize Their Recurrence Are Not Compatible with Each Other. How Should We Approach Prevention of Future Uroliths?

Answer: Please refer to the article entitled, "Changing Paradigms in Compound Uroliths" in this edition of Veterinary Clinics of North America for information about this problem.

37. What Urolith Types Are Most Commonly Found in Young Dogs?

Answer: Between 1981 and 2002, 2102 uroliths from dogs less than 1 year of age were analyzed at the Minnesota Urolith Center. 56% were struvite, 22% were purine, 5% were calcium oxalate, 2% were calcium phosphate, and 2% were cystine. Infection-induced struvite is the most common cause of uroliths in immature dogs. Urate stones associated with portovascular shunts are also common. Reference #1, osborne, lulich, polzin et al. Analysis of 77000 urolith. VCNA.

38. The Dog Previously Had Struvite Uroliths and Now Has Calcium Oxalate Crystals or Uroliths. How Is This Possible?

Answer: Sometimes calcium oxalate uroliths form following successful management preventing struvite uroliths and vice versa. Sometime uroliths contain both struvite and calcium oxalate. The dilemma is how to manage both of these mineral types. We recommend that emphasis be placed on minimizing the recurrence of calcium oxalate uroliths since they cannot be dissolved medically.[17]

39. How Often Are Uroliths Overlooked in the Urinary Tract During Surgery?

Answer: In a retrospective study, urocystoliths were detected in the lower urinary tract of 15% to 20% of dogs and cats immediately following cystotomy.[18] If the number of uroliths present in the urinary tract can be accurately determined by survey or contrast radiography, it is usually unnecessary to obtain immediate postsurgical films to ensure that they have all been removed since they can be accurately counted. However, if the numbers of uroliths detected by radiography are too numerous to count, postsurgical radiographs are indicated to detect uroliths that have been inadvertently allowed to remain in the urinary tract.[15] Results of quantitative analysis on the retrieved uroliths will determine the best management protocol for any stones remaining in the urinary tract.

40. Radiographic Evaluation of a Dog's Coxofemoral Joints for Evidence of Arthritis Reveals Two Small Uroliths in the Bladder. Should They Be Removed?

Answer: Not always. If uroliths are detected in the bladder and the patient is asymptomatic without significant bacteriuria, the option to monitor the urolith activity is an alternative to surgery. However, the owner should be informed that the patient may be at increased risk for urinary tract infection or urethral obstruction, and instructed to monitor the patient accordingly.[19] Depending on the mineral type, medical dissolution may also be an option.

41. What Is the Best Method to Manage Nephroliths?

Answer: Because of the risk of surgical damage to functional kidney tissue during surgery, if the nephroliths are presumed to be calcium oxalate and not associated with obstruction of urine flow, uncontrollable infection, or deterioration of renal function, monitoring kidney stone activity and selecting protocols to minimize urolith growth may be the best course of action. Monitor the status of the patient's nephrolith activity by radiography or ultrasonography every two to six months, unless clinical signs mandate more frequent evaluation.[17]

UROLITH RECURRENCE
42. How Quickly Can the Uroliths Reform? Will They Recur?

Answer: Urolith formation is a process that typically takes several weeks (eg, infection-induced struvite) to months (eg, calcium oxalate) rather than days. A retrospective study looking at 438 dogs, with a variety of urolith types, found a recurrence rate of 25%.[20]

Struvite: Infection-induced uroliths can form within a few days to a few weeks following infection of the urinary tract with urease-producing microbes. Struvite uroliths associated with urinary tract infections (UTI) caused by *Staphylococci* or *Proteus spp* have been detected in puppies as young as five weeks of age.[21]

Calcium oxalate: Thirty-three calcium oxalate–forming dogs were evaluated for recurrent uroliths by postsurgical radiography following surgical removal of uroliths. Radiographs evaluated immediately following surgery confirmed that all uroliths were removed. After one year, uroliths were detected by radiography or urolith retrieval in 36% of the dogs. After 2 years, the recurrence rate was 42%, and after 3 years it was 48%. The diet and therapy these patients were receiving, if any, was not specified.[22]

Purine: Purine uroliths appear to have a high recurrence rate. A retrospective study of 438 dogs revealed a minimum recurrence rate of 33%.[20]

Cystine: Because cystinuria is an inherited metabolic defect, uroliths frequently recur within 2 to 12 months.[23]

43. Uroliths Were Detected in the Urinary Tract by Postsurgical Radiography. How Should I Proceed?

Answer: If small uroliths are detected on postoperative films, they may be removed nonsurgically either by catheter retrieval or voiding urohydropropulsion after healing of the bladder occurs.[24] If the analysis results indicate that the uroliths removed are cystine, struvite, or urate, it may be possible to dissolve the remaining uroliths with diet and medical therapy.

44. The Uroliths Have Recurred. Is Surgery the Only Option for Removal?

Answer: If the recurrent uroliths are small enough, they may be removed by minimally invasive techniques (ie, catheter retrieval or voiding urohydropropulsion).[24] If it is suspected that the uroliths are struvite, urate, or cystine; dietary and medication therapy can be used in an effort to dissolve the uroliths. If the patient is asymptomatic one option to consider is initiating therapy to minimize urolith growth. Intracorporeal lithotripsy may be considered for urethroliths. Surgery is an option for urolith removal if the recurrent uroliths become problematic.

45. Postsurgical Films Did Not Indicate Any Uroliths, But Radiographs of the Entire Urinary Tract Obtained 4 Weeks Postsurgery Revealed Several Small Uroliths in the Bladder Lumen. How Is This Possible?

Answer: Uroliths on postsurgical radiographs can be missed due to a variety of reasons including:

- Overexposure of radiographs.
- Error in patient positioning.
- Portions of the urinary tract obscured by the pelvis.
- Air in bladder lumen or abdominal cavity following surgery.

In some patients, infection-induced struvite urolith can recur during this short period of time. Other urolith types generally take longer to recur and are so small at 4 weeks that they are not detectible by routine radiographs.[25]

URINALYSIS
46. What Is a Normal Urine pH for a Dog Or for a Cat?

Answer: Urine pH for dogs and cats typically falls within a range of 5.5 to 7.5 pH units, but on occasion may be slightly higher or lower.[26]

47. What Is the Best Time To Collect a Urine Sample: Fasted Or Postprandial?

Answer: Both. For routine screening, samples may be collected at any time. There are advantages for collecting urine during specific periods of the day. Early morning samples are preferred to evaluate normal dogs and cats, since these samples are more likely to be concentrated and more likely to be acidic. Acidity tends to prevent dissolution of proteinaceous structures, such as cells and casts.[27] Postprandial urine samples collected 3 to 6 hours after eating may be used to evaluate the effect of diet on urine pH, specific gravity and crystalluria.[27]

48. Is Refrigeration the Best Way to Preserve Urine Following Collection?

Answer: Refrigeration is a method of preservation for urine samples that cannot be analyzed within 30 to 60 minutes following collection. It is often preferred over other methods of chemical preservation that may interfere with reagent strip tests. Unfortunately, the change in temperature associated with refrigeration is a common cause of in vitro crystalluria.[28] Therefore, detection of crystals in refrigerated samples should be validated by reevaluation of fresh urine. If a sample has been refrigerated, ideally it should be allowed to return to room temperature before analysis.

49. How Useful Are pH Meters in Evaluation of Urine?

Answer: Because accurate and consistent urine pH values are important in monitoring patients with uroliths, we recommend monitoring the patient's urine with a portable pH meter. Urine pH values obtained by reagent strips (colorimetric dyes) may vary by as much as 0.5 units on either side of the observed value. A recent study comparing portable (handheld) pH meters, reagent test strips, and pH indicator paper strips indicated that inexpensive portable pH meters correlated well with values obtained with expensive benchtop pH meter models.[29]

50. How Often Should I Monitor Urinalysis?

Answer: Monitor the urine frequently during initial stages of evaluation. How frequently is somewhat dependent on the type of urolith the patient had and how quickly the uroliths can form. By monitoring the urine you can determine if changes in the diet or medical treatment are warranted. In patients with rapidly recurring uroliths, such as struvite, cystine, and urate, urine should be monitored weekly to determine if therapy is effective. Once efficacy is established, urine may be evaluated every 2 to 4 weeks depending on the needs of the patient. For slower recurring uroliths such as calcium oxalate and silica, monitor every 4 weeks, then intervals between follow-up examinations may be approximately every 3 months. Remember early detection of recurrence may allow use of nonsurgical techniques for removal such as voiding urohydropulsion or catheter retrieval.[24]

51. The Patient's Owner Has Been Feeding the Recommended Diet; However, Persistent Crystalluria Has Been Occurring. Why Is This Happening?

Answer: The detection of crystals in urine indicates that the sample is oversaturated with crystalline substances. This may occur as a result of in vitro or in vivo events. Fresh urine samples should be analyzed as soon after collection as possible to verify that in vivo crystalluria is significant. Monitoring the patient's urine pH, specific gravity, and serum urea nitrogen values should be considered to evaluate owner and patient compliance and the effectiveness and safety of therapy. If the patient's lab values are not in the expected range, the probability that she or he is eating something in addition to, or instead of, the recommended diet should be discussed, preferably with the person responsible for the care of the animal. For example, dogs eating a low-protein canned diet such as Hill's u/d should have a urine specific gravity of <1.020 and a serum urea nitrogen of <1.7 nmol/L.[30]

52. Why Is the Urine pH Higher or Lower than Expected?

Answer: If the urine pH is not what is expected, ask the owner if they are feeding the recommended diet or if they are adding additional food treats. Patients eating a diet high in fruits, legumes, and vegetables tend to have more alkaline urine; and those eating diets high in protein tend to form more acidic urine. If the patient has a urinary tract infection with urease producing bacteria, prolonged time between collection and analysis of unpreserved samples allow the bacteria to alter the urine and make it more alkaline. Often lack of owner compliance is a key reason why the urine pH or specific gravity are not what you expect.

53. We Rechecked the Dog's Urine and Found that It Has Calcium Oxalate and Struvite Crystals in the Same Urine Sediment Sample. Is There a Plausible Explanation for This Observation?

Answer: Additional information is required to provide a meaningful answer:

How was the sample collected? Cystocentesis is the ideal method to collect urine for analysis, especially when monitoring a patient for recurrent infections.

How much time lapsed between collection and analysis? This information may be helpful in determining if the crystals are in vitro artifacts.

Was there a significant number of bacteria in the urine? In properly collected and preserved urine samples, struvite crystals are often significant when they are observed in association with bacteria and white cells.

Was the urine sample refrigerated? Refrigeration of urine could promote in vitro calcium oxalate crystalluria in a urine sample with in vivo struvite crystalluria.[28]

54. Why Do We Need to Perform Urinalyses In-House?

Answer: When performing routine urinalyses, it is acceptable to send urine samples to a reputable clinical pathology laboratory. But when monitoring a patient with a history of urolithiasis, perform the urinalysis in-house as soon after collection as possible to minimize in vitro changes in the sample.

DIETS
55. What Diet Should I Feed While I Wait for the Results of Urolith Analysis?

Answer: Feed a diet unlikely to enhance urolith formation that avoids mineral excesses or deficits. The diet should also promote a neutral urine pH. If possible, feed a canned diet to reduce urine concentration. Once the results of the urolith analysis are received, follow the appropriate recommendation protocols to promote dissolution or minimize recurrence. Specific recommendations for each mineral type can be found at the Center's Web site.

56. I Have Received the Results of Urolith Analysis, Which Diet Should I Consider?

Answer: Uroliths form when urine is oversaturated with one or more lithogenic components. The goal of management is to correct as many risk factors as possible (eg, urinary tract infections caused by urease producing microbes; reduce hyperammonemia and hyperuricemia, etc). Several dietary risk factors may contribute to oversaturation; therefore, reducing urine concentration by feeding a canned diet is a common recommendation for prevention of all mineral types of stones. Due to the increasing variety of manufacturers that make therapeutic diets to prevent urolith recurrence, we recommend that you contact diet manufacturers directly to determine the quality of evidence available to support their recommendations, and to determine if any of their manufactured diets meets your patient's needs.

57. How Strict Does Dietary Compliance Have to Be?

Answer: Veterinarians and their staff frequently overestimate the degree to which clients comply with management recommendations. To enhance compliance, clients should be included in the planning so that the prevention protocol includes what they can do, and excludes what they cannot or will not do. Educating clients about the expected benefits associated with therapy, and the expected adverse outcomes if therapy is not implemented enhances compliance. Therapy requiring changes in lifestyle (eg, meal feeding versus ad libitum feeding), confusion about instructions, too many medications, and difficult tasks (eg, frequent oral administration of pills to cats) are likely to reduce compliance. However, an expectation of full compliance is often unrealistic. In general, less than full compliance is acceptable as long as the desired therapeutic benefit can safely be achieved.[16]

58. Should I Feed a Canned or Dry Food?

Answer: One of our goals in urolith prevention is to promote a less concentrated urine (urine specific gravity <1.020). We recommend feeding canned diets, which are approximately 70% to 80% moisture, to dogs and cats with a history of urolithiasis.

59. My Dog or Cat Does Not Like Eating Canned Diets. What Are Your Recommendations?

Answer: While we all think pets should love eating a canned diet after years of eating dry food, we are often surprised to see them turn up their noses at canned food. Try warming the food slightly (be sure that it is not too hot) to enhance palatability of the food. If necessary, instruct the owner to make the change from the patient's current diet to the recommended food very slowly. Sometimes pets are very resistant to change, and by making the change over several days (7–14 days) they may accept the new diet. Try adding flavor-enhanced water to the canned food or add water to the dry food. Monitor the patient's urine frequently and aim for a urine with a specific gravity of 1.020 or less. Remember, if a patient is currently sick, it is best not to change the food until they are feeling better, to avoid a negative food association (food aversion).

60. Are There Any Resources That I Can Rely Upon to Evaluate the Safety and Efficacy of Homemade Diets?

Answer: Several text books and Web sites provide recommendations for homemade diets designed to promote urolith dissolution and to minimize recurrence of various types of uroliths. Since urolith-formers may have other conditions such as food allergies, diabetes, etc. that are best managed by dietary changes contrary to those recommended to minimize urolith recurrence, it may not be possible to find a manufactured diet that will optimally meet your patient's needs. Veterinary nutritionists are available to formulate a diet that best meets the patient's needs. Many veterinary colleges or veterinary specialty centers have a veterinary nutritionist on staff. Access to veterinary nutritionists also may be obtained from various websites.

61. Can I Use Over-The-Counter Dog Foods to Manage the Urinary Issues?

Answer: With the exception of infection-induced canine struvite, we do not have experience using over-the-counter-diets to minimize urolith recurrence. Infection-induced canine struvite can be prevented by eradicating and controlling bacterial infections of the urinary tract. Although a therapeutic diet in combination with an antimicrobic is required to dissolve infection-induced struvite uroliths, infection-induced struvite will not recur unless there is a UTI caused by urease producing microbes. Provided that the infection is eradicated or controlled, a complete and balanced canned over-the-counter grocery brand diet that meets NRC recommendations should be satisfactory to prevent recurrence in infection-induced struvite patients. The patient should be monitored for recurrent UTI and struvite uroliths at appropriate intervals.

62. How Do I Convince the Pet Owner to Feed the Recommended Product?

Answer: Sometimes due to financial reasons pet owners cannot afford to feed a therapeutic diet. Others prefer a homemade diet or are resistant to change. The veterinarian and owner in partnership need to work toward finding the best diet or medical therapy to help reduce the risk of recurrence within the owner's desires and financial limitations.

63. Can I Mix Other Foods with a Urolith-Management Food to Treat Multiple Problems?

Answer: It is difficult to answer the question without knowing what problems you are attempting to treat. If an alkalinizing diet is being fed and mixed with an acidifying diet the combination would likely eliminate the desired effect of both diets. In most situations it would be best to find a diet that is designed to manage the problem of greatest significance.

64. What Treats Can I Feed While Trying to Prevent Struvite, Calcium Oxalate, Cystine, Urate Uroliths?

Answer: In patients with a history of struvite uroliths, control and prevention of urinary tract infections is the primary means of preventing further urolith recurrence. Feeding small quantities of treats should not contribute to the recurrence of this urolith type.

For other urolith types, the decision to give treats should be based on the ingredients, and the mineral type of the urolith retrieved from the dog. Evidence derived from retrospective case-control studies of risk factors associated with calcium oxalate urolithiasis in dogs revealed that dogs fed substantial quantities of manufactured dietary treats were up to 5 times more likely to develop calcium oxalate uroliths then dogs not fed treats (Lekcharoensuk C, unpublished data, 2001). Many owners give their dogs human foods as treats. A list of human foods that are acceptable, and foods to avoid, when attempting to minimize formation or recurrence of calcium oxalate and urate uroliths has been extrapolated from reports about urolithiasis in humans.[31,32] Evidence derived from a retrospective case-control study evaluating environmental risk factors associated with calcium oxalate urolithiasis in dogs revealed when the daily allowance of human food fed a dogs was $\geq 1/8$ of the total, the risk of calcium oxalate urolith formation was 14% greater compared with dogs whose diets contain less than one-eighth of human food (Lekcharoensuk C, unpublished data, 2001). Since it is recommended that the owner feed a canned diet for prevention, small amounts of the dry formula can be used as treats.

WATER
65. How Do I Get the Patient to Drink More Water?

Answer: There are several options to encourage a patient to consume more water:

- Use a pet water fountain to provide continuous filtered fresh running water.
- Provide the pet with fresh water in water dishes located in multiple sites.
- Add a small amount of flavoring agent to drinking water such as tuna juice or low-sodium bouillon.
- Add additional water to dry or wet food.
- Offer the dog or cat ice cubes as additional fluid and as a treat.

66. Why Is the Recommendation to Drink Adequate Amounts of Fluid Important?

Answer: An excessive concentration of minerals or crystals in the urine is a prerequisite for urolith formation. Therefore, increased water intake has at least two beneficial outcomes. First, it leads to the dilution of crystalline material in the urine, and second, it reduces the risk of recurrence because the formation of large volumes of urine increases the frequency of micturition and the frequency that crystals will be voided.[33]

67. How Can One Assess Whether Or Not the Patient Is Drinking Adequate Quantities of Fluid?

Answer: The easiest way to monitor the amount of fluid that a patient is drinking is to measure the specific gravity of the urine. The goal is to try and maintain a urine specific gravity of less than 1.020.

68. Is Hard Water a Risk Factor For Urolithiasis? Should I Give Distilled Water?

Answer: In general, increasing water intake with the goal of decreasing urine concentration and increasing urine volume should be considered as a key component of medical management for all types of uroliths. A retrospective case-control study designed to evaluate risk factors associated with calcium oxalate urolithiasis in dogs revealed that when well water was the primary source of drinking water, the risk for calcium oxalate was reduced by 41%. However, these results may be confounded by other factors indicating that a reduced risk of calcium oxalate had also been observed in dogs living in a rural environment (Lekcharoensuk C, unpublished data, 2001). A study of cats did not reveal that the source of water was associated with calcium oxalate urolith formation.[34] It is unlikely that water hardness plays a significant role in the formation of uroliths. The quantity of water consumed is much more important. Use of distilled water is of questionable value unless its flavor enhances water consumption.

MISCELLANEOUS
69. Can We Give Rawhide Chews?

Answer: We have not studied the effect of this type of treat as it relates to the dissolution and or prevention of uroliths. However, since rawhide chews are made of approximately 60%–80% low-quality protein, we do not recommend feeding them to patients when eating a high protein diet is contraindicated.

70. Are Glucosamine Supplements Beneficial?

Answer: The use of glucosamine supplements in urolith patients is probably not harmful. Some investigators indicate that glucosamine use may be helpful in inhibiting calcium oxalate crystal adherence to the bladder wall. However, we have not studied the effects of glucosamine as it relates to the dissolution and or prevention of uroliths.

71. What About Toothpaste or Toothbrushing?

Answer: We have no studies to evaluate the effects of toothpaste and urolith recurrence. Given the small quantity of toothpaste likely to be consumed, we hypothesize that it would have no effect on the status of urolithiasis.

REFERENCES

1. Osborne CA, Lulich JP, Polzin DJ, et al. Analysis of 77,000 canine uroliths: perspectives from the Minnesota Urolith Center. Vet Clin North Am Small Anim Pract 1999;29(1):17–38.
2. Osborne CA, Clinton CW, Moran HC, et al. Comparison of qualitative and quantitative analyses of canine uroliths. Vet Clin North Am Small Anim Pract 1986; 16(2):317–23.

3. Safranow K, Machoy Z, Ciechanowski K. Analysis of purines in urinary calculi by high-performance liquid chromatography. Anal Biochem 2000;286(Issue 2): 224–30.
4. Osborne CA, Lulich JP, Polzin DJ, et al. Medical dissolution and prevention of canine struvite urolithiasis. Twenty years of experience. Vet Clin North Am Small Anim Pract 1999;29(1):73–111.
5. Koide T, Itatani H, Yoshioka T, et al. Clinical manifestations of calcium oxalate monohydrate and dihydrate urolithiasis. J Urol 1982;127:1067–9.
6. Leusmann DB, Meyer-Jurgens UB, Kleinhans G. Scanning electron microscopy of urinary calculi: some peculiarities. Scan Electron Microsc 1984;3:1427–32.
7. Otnes B. Urinary stone analysis: methods, materials and value. Scand J Urol Nephrol 1983;71(Suppl):1–109.
8. Schubert G, Brien G. Crystallographic investigations of urinary calcium oxalate calculi. Int J Urol Nephrol 1981;13:249–60.
9. Tomazic BB, Nancollas GH. The dissolution of calcium oxalate kidney stones: a kinetic study. J Urol 1982;128:205–8.
10. Berenyl M, Frang D, Legrady J. Theoretical and clinical importance of the differentiation between the two types of calcium oxalate hydrate. Int J Urol Nephrol 1972;4:341–5.
11. Osborne CA. How would you manage feline xanthine urocystoliths? DVM Newsmagazine, May 1, 2003.
12. van Zuilen CD, Nickel RF, van Dijk TN, et al. Xanthinuria in a family of Cavalier King charles spaniels. Vet Q 1997;19(4):172–4.
13. Bartges JW, Osborne CA, Felice LJ, et al. Influence of allopurinol and two diets on 24-hour urinary excretions of uric acid, xanthine, and ammonia by healthy dogs. Am J Vet Res 1995;56:595–9.
14. Osborne CA. How would you manage cystine urocystoliths in a female Siamese cat? DVM Newsmagazine, Feb 1, 2003.
15. Osborne CA. Improving management of urolithiasis: diagnostic caveats. DVM Newsmagazine, Jan 1, 2004.
16. Osborne CA. Improving management of urolithiasis: therapeutic caveats. DVM Newsmagazine, Feb 1, 2004.
17. Lulich JP, Osborne CA, Lekcharoensuk C, et al. Canine calcium oxalate urolithiasis: case-based applications of therapeutic principles. Vet Clin North Am Small Anim Pract 1999;29(1):123–39.
18. Lulich JP, Osborne CA, Polzin JP, et al. Incomplete removal of canine and feline urocystoliths by cystotomy. Proc 11th ACVIM Forum; Washington, DC May 1993. p. 932.
19. Osborne CA, Finco DR. Canine and Feline Nephrology and Urology. Canine and feline urolithiases: relationship of etiopathogenesis to treatment and prevention. Williams and Wikins; 1995. p. 814.
20. Brown NO, Parks JL, Greene RW. Recurrence of canine urolithiasis, JAVMA 170(4): Feb 15, 1977, 419–22.
21. Osborne CA. Improving management of urolithiasis: canine struvite uroliths. DVM Newsmagazine, April 1, 2004.
22. Lulich JP, Perrine L, Osborne CA, et al. Postsurgical recurrence of calcium oxalate uroliths in dogs. ACVIM Abstract 1992;vol. 6(2):119.
23. Osborne CA, Sanderson SL, Lulich JP, et al. Canine cystine urolithiasis: cause, detection, treatment, and prevention. Vet Clin North Am Small Anim Pract 1999;29(1): 193–211.

24. Lulich JP, Osborne CA, Sanderson SL, et al. Voiding urohydropropulsion: lessons from 5 years of experience. In: Veterinary Clinics of North America Small Animal Practice, 29. Philadelphia: WB Saunders; 1999. p. 283–92.
25. Weichselbaum RC, Feeney DA, Jessen CR, et al. Urocystolith detection: comparison survey, contrast radiographic and ultrasonographic techniques in an in vitro bladder phantom. Vet Radiol Ultrasound 1999;40:386–400.
26. Osborne CA, Stevens JB. Biochemical analysis of urine: indications, methods, interpretation. In: Osborne CA, Stevens JB, editors. Urinalysis: guide to compassionate patient care. Shawnee Mission (KS): Bayer Co.; 1999. p. 87–124.
27. Osborne CA, Stevens JB. "Prophet"-ing more from urinalysis: maximizing reproducible test results. In: Osborne CA, Stevens JB, editors. Urinalysis: guide to compassionate patient care. Shawnee Mission (KS): Bayer Co.; 1999. p. 51–63.
28. Albasan H, Lulich JP, Osborne CA, et al. Effects of storage time and temperature on pH, specific gravity, and crystal formation in urine samples from dogs and cats. J Am Vet Med Assoc 2003;vol. 222(2):176–9.
29. Johnson KY, Lulich JP, Osborne CA. Evaluation of the reproducibility and accuracy of pH-determining devices used to measure urine pH in dogs. J Am Vet Med Assoc 2007;vol. 230(3):364–9.
30. Hills key to clinical nutrition. Hill's Pet Nutrition, Inc.; 2007. p. 90.
31. Osborne CA, Lulich JP, Bartges JW. The ROCKet Science of canine urolithiasis. Vet Clin North Am Small Anim Pract, January 1999; Vol 29, no 1.
32. Pak, CYC. Renal stone disease: pathogenesis, prevention, and treatment. Boston: Martinus Nijhoff Publishing; 1987.
33. Osborne CA. How to simplify management of complex uroliths. DVM Newsmagazine, September 1, 2003.
34. Kirk CA, Ling GV, Franti CE, et al. Evaluation of factors associated with development of calcium oxalate urolithiasis in cats. J Am Vet Med Assoc 1995;vol. 207(11):1429–34.

Analysis of 451,891 Canine Uroliths, Feline Uroliths, and Feline Urethral Plugs from 1981 to 2007: Perspectives from the Minnesota Urolith Center

Carl A. Osborne, DVM, PhD[a],*, Jody P. Lulich, DVM, PhD[a],
John M. Kruger, DVM, PhD[b], Lisa K. Ulrich, CVT[a], Lori A. Koehler, CVT[a]

KEYWORDS
- Urolith • Calculi • Stone • Urolith analyisi • Urethral plug
- Urolith trends

Urolithiasis is a general term referring to the causes and effects of stones anywhere in the urinary tract. Urolithiasis should not be viewed conceptually as a single disease with a single cause, but rather as a sequela of multiple interacting underlying abnormalities. Thus, the syndrome of urolithiasis may be defined as the occurrence of familial, congenital, or acquired pathophysiologic factors that, in combination, progressively increase the risk of precipitation of excretory metabolites in urine to form stones (ie, uroliths).

With the support of an Educational Grant from Hill's Pet Nutrition, the Minnesota Urolith Center (MUC) has performed quantitative analysis of uroliths retrieved from animals for more than 2.5 decades. During this period, the authors have observed dramatic shifts in urolith type. The following epidemiologic discussion is based on quantitative analysis of 350,803 canine uroliths (**Figs. 1–3**, **Tables 1** and **2**), 94,778 feline uroliths (**Figs. 4–6**, **Tables 3** and **4**), and 6,310 feline urethral plugs (**Figs. 7–9**, **Tables 5** and **6**) submitted to the MUC from 1981 to 2007.

[a] Veterinary Clinical Sciences Department, Minnesota Urolith Center, College of Veterinary Medicine, University of Minnesota, 1352 Boyd Avenue, St. Paul, MN 55108, USA
[b] Department of Small Animal Clinical Sciences, Michigan State University College of Veterinary Medicine, Room D208, Veterinary Teaching Hospital, East Lansing, MI 48824-1314, USA
* Corresponding author.
E-mail address: osbor002@umn.edu (C.A. Osborne).

Vet Clin Small Anim 39 (2008) 183–197
doi:10.1016/j.cvsm.2008.09.011
0195-5616/08/$ – see front matter © 2008 Elsevier Inc. All rights reserved.
vetsmall.theclinics.com

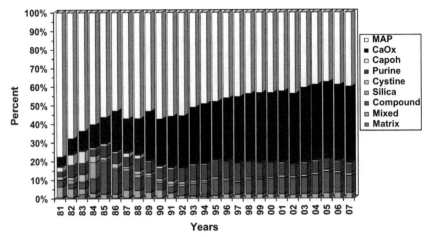

Fig. 1. Canine urolith distribution: 1981 to 2007.

EPIDEMIOLOGY OF CANINE UROLITHS

In 1981, calcium oxalate was detected in only 5% of canine uroliths submitted to the MUC, whereas struvite (magnesium ammonium phosphate or MAP) was detected in 78%. However, evaluation of the prevalence of different types of minerals in canine uroliths during successive years revealed a gradual and consistent increase in occurrence of calcium oxalate uroliths, and a gradual and consistent decline in the occurrence of struvite uroliths (see **Fig. 1**). In fact, by 2003 the prevalence of calcium oxalate (41%) was approximately equal to struvite (40%). In 2004, calcium oxalate (41%) surpassed struvite (39%). In 2005, calcium oxalate was detected in 42% of the urolith submissions, while struvite was detected in (38%). In 2006, calcium oxalate was again detected in 41% of the canine urolith submissions, while struvite was detected in 39%. In 2007, 40% of the urolith submissions were struvite while calcium oxalate represented 41% (see **Fig. 3** and **Table 2**). The total submission ($n = 40{,}612$) of canine uroliths in 2007 was 4,580 more than for the year 2006 ($n = 36{,}032$).

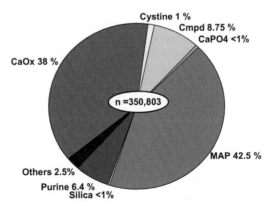

Fig. 2. Mineral composition of canine uroliths: 1981 to 2007.

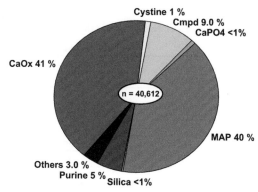

Cystine 1 %
Cmpd 9.0 %
CaPO4 <1%

CaOx 41 %

n = 40,612

MAP 40 %

Others 3.0 %
Purine 5 % Silica <1%

Fig. 3. Mineral composition of canine uroliths 2007.

EPIDEMIOLOGY OF FELINE UROLITHS

The change in frequency of feline calcium oxalate and struvite occurrence was even more dramatic than the occurrence of canine struvite and calcium oxalate uroliths during a similar period. In 1981, calcium oxalate was detected in only 2% of feline uroliths submitted to the MUC, whereas struvite was detected in 78% (see **Fig. 4**). However, beginning in the mid-1980s, a dramatic increase in the frequency of calcium oxalate uroliths occurred in association with a decrease in the frequency of struvite uroliths. In 2002, approximately 55% of the feline uroliths submitted to the MUC were composed of calcium oxalate, while only 33% were composed of struvite. During this

Table 1
Mineral composition[a] of 350,803 canine uroliths evaluated at the MUC from 1981 to 2007

Struvite	149,199	42.5%
Magnesium hydrogen phosphate	52	0.01%
Magnesium phosphate hydrate	4	<0.01%
Calcium oxalate	133,338	38.0%
Calcium phosphate	1801	0.5%
Purines	22,412	6.4%
Cystine	3402	1.0%
Silica	1414	0.4%
Calcium carbonate	6	<0.01%
Dolomite	1	<0.01%
Mixed[b]	8146	2.3%
Compound[c]	30,832	8.8%
Matrix	153	0.04%
Drug metabolite	19	<0.01
Other	24	<0.01
Total	350,803	100%

[a] Analyzed by polarizing light microscopy or infrared spectroscopy.
[b] Uroliths did not contain at least 70% of mineral type listed; no nucleus or shell detected.
[c] Uroliths contained an identifiable nucleus and one or more surrounding layers of a different mineral type.

Table 2
Mineral composition[a] of 40,612 canine uroliths evaluated at the MUC, 2007

Predominant Mineral Type	Number of Uroliths	%
Magnesium ammonium phosphate $6H_2O$	16,124	39
Magnesium hydrogen phosphate $3H_2O$	5	0.01
Magnesium phosphate hydrate	1	<0.1
Calcium oxalate	16,761	41.3
Calcium phosphate	273	0.7
Purines	2,020	5.0
Xanthine	43	0.1
Cystine	447	1.1
Silica	134	0.3
Other	1	<0.1
Calcium carbonate	2	<0.1
Mixed[b]	1,132	2.8
Compound[c]	3,698	9.1
Matrix	10	<0.1
Drug metabolite	4	<0.1
Date 2007	40,612	100

[a] Analyzed by polarizing light microscopy or infrared spectroscopy.
[b] Uroliths did not contain at least 70% of mineral type listed; no nucleus or shell detected.
[c] Uroliths contained an identifiable nucleus and one or more surrounding layers of a different mineral type.

period, the decline in appearance of naturally occurring struvite uroliths associated with a reciprocal increase in calcium oxalate uroliths may have been associated with: (1) the widespread use of a calculolytic diet designed to dissolve struvite uroliths; (2) modification of maintenance and prevention diets to minimize struvite crystalluria (some dietary risk factors that decrease the risk of struvite uroliths increase the risk of calcium oxalate uroliths); and (3) inconsistent follow-up evaluation of efficacy of dietary management protocols by urinalysis and radiography.

In 2003, the trends in the occurrence in feline uroliths began to change again. The frequency of feline calcium oxalate uroliths declined to 47%, while the frequency of struvite uroliths increased to 42% (see **Fig. 4**). During 2004, the number of struvite uroliths (44.9%) submitted to the MUC nudged past those containing calcium oxalate (44.3%). In 2005, the number of struvite uroliths (48.1%) surpassed those containing calcium oxalate (40.6%) in frequency of occurrence (see **Fig. 6**). Of 10,093 feline uroliths submitted to the MUC in 2006, 5,001 (50%) were struvite and 3,914 (39%) were calcium oxalate. In 2007, of 11,174 uroliths submitted to the MUC, 5,432 (49%) were struvite, and 4,553 (41%) were calcium oxalate (see **Figs. 4** and **6, Tables 3** and **4**). The progressive decrease in occurrence of naturally occurring calcium oxalate uroliths during the past 5 years may be associated with reformulation of adult maintenance diets to minimize risk factors for calcium oxalate crystalluria, improvements in formulation of therapeutic diets designed to reduce risk factors for calcium oxalate uroliths, and increased use of therapeutic diets designed to reduce risk factors for calcium oxalate uroliths. The increase in appearance of naturally occurring struvite uroliths during the past 5 years may be associated with the reciprocal relationship between some dietary risk factors for calcium oxalate and struvite uroliths.[1,2] For example, diets that reduce urine acidity and provide adequate quantities of magnesium reduce the risk of

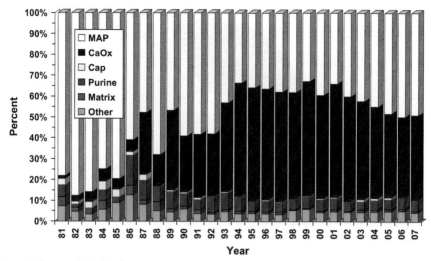

Fig. 4. Feline urolith distribution: 1981–2007.

calcium oxalate urolith formation, but increase the risk of struvite (magnesium ammonium phosphate) urolith formation. Whatever the reasons, it is likely that most of the 5,432 sterile struvite uroliths retrieved from cats and submitted to the MUC in 2007 could have been readily dissolved in 2 to 4 weeks by feeding a diet designed to promote formation of urine that is undersaturated with struvite.[3]

EPIDEMIOLOGY OF FELNE URETHRAL PLUGS

The team at the MUC has emphasized differences in the structure and composition between uroliths and urethral plugs.[4] Urethral plugs contain varying quantities of minerals in proportion to large quantities of matrix (**Figs. 10–13**).

What would be an estimate of the occurrence of feline calcium oxalate urethral plug submissions to the MUC from 1981to 2007? Unlike feline and canine stones, since 1981 struvite has consistently been the most common mineral identified in urethral plugs (see **Figs. 7–9**, **Tables 5** and **6**). The prevalence of calcium oxalate in urethral plugs always has been infrequent. Of 506 urethral plugs submitted to the MUC by veterinarians in

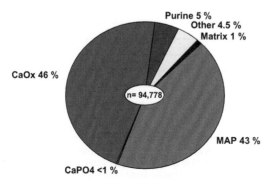

Fig. 5. Mineral composition of feline uroliths 1981–2007.

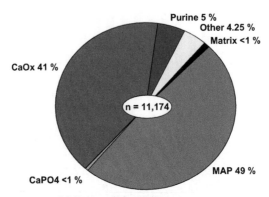

Fig. 6. Mineral composition of feline uroliths 2007.

2007, the mineral composition of approximately 92% was primarily struvite. Approximately 1% were composed of calcium oxalate (see **Fig. 9** and **Table 6**).

The explanation as to why there have been significant shifts in the prevalence of calcium oxalate and struvite in feline uroliths during the past 25 years, while the prevalence of struvite and calcium oxalate in feline urethral plugs has not significantly changed, is not obvious. During the same time, the mineral composition of other types of uroliths has been associated with no obvious trend (see **Figs. 1, 4** and **7; Tables 1, 3,** and **5**).

In a retrospective study of approximately 1,000 feline calcium oxalate uroliths evaluated at the MUC, only 3 were formed by cats less than 1 year of age.[5] Of the cats affected with calcium oxalate uroliths, 97% were greater than 2 years of age. The greatest risk for developing calcium oxalate uroliths occurred in 10- to 15-year-old neutered male cats. These observations are of interest because it has been

Table 3
Mineral composition[a] of 94,776 feline uroliths evaluated at the MUC from 1981 to 2007

Predominant Mineral Type	Number	%
Struvite	40,554	42.8
Magnesium hydrogen phosphate	93	0.1
Magnesium phosphate hydrate	189	0.2
Calcium oxalate	43,707	46.1
Calcium phosphate	338	0.4
Cystine	92	0.1
Silica	41	<0.1
Mixed[b]	928	1.0
Compound[c]	3,135	3.3
Matrix	925	1.0
Drug metabolite	5	0.0
Other	56	0.1
Total	94,776	100

[a] Analyzed by polarizing light microscopy or infrared spectroscopy.
[b] Uroliths did not contain at least 70% of mineral type listed; no nucleus or shell detected.
[c] Uroliths contained an identifiable nucleus and one or more surrounding layers of a different mineral type.

Table 4
Mineral composition[a] of 11,174 feline uroliths evaluated at the MUC, 2007

Predominant Mineral Type	Number of Uroliths	%
Magnesium ammonium phosphate 6H_2O	5,432	48.6
Magnesium hydrogen phosphate 3H_2O	7	0.06
Magnesium phosphate hydrate	42	0.38
Calcium oxalate	4,553	40.8
Calcium phosphate	30	0.3
Purines	523	4.9
Xanthine	27	<0.1
Cystine	12	<0.1
Silica	8	<0.1
Other	10	<0.1
Mixed[b]	81	0.7
Compound[c]	356	3.2
Matrix	93	0.8
Date 2007	11,174	100

[a] Analyzed by polarizing light microscopy or infrared spectroscopy.
[b] Uroliths did not contain at least 70% of mineral type listed; no nucleus or shell detected.
[c] Uroliths contained an identifiable nucleus and one or more surrounding layers of a different mineral type.

hypothesized that conditions promoting urine acidity are a risk factor for calcium oxalate urolithiasis. It has been reported however, that the urine pH of young cats is lower than that of adults consuming the same diet.[6] One explanation advanced to explain this phenomenon is that growing animals synthesize bone mineral from calcium and phosphate in the blood. Phosphate circulates in the blood as HPO_4^{-2} and

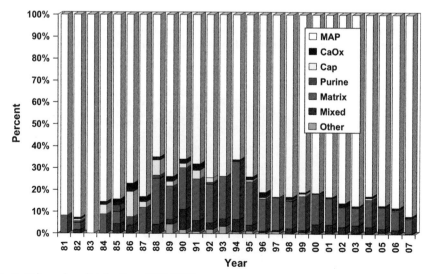

Fig. 7. Feline plug distribution: 1981–2007.

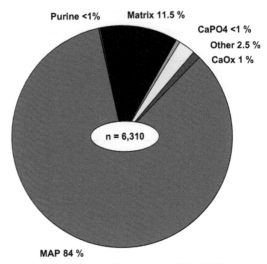

Purine <1%   Matrix 11.5 %

CaPO4 <1 %
Other 2.5 %
CaOx 1 %

n = 6,310

MAP 84 %

Fig. 8. Mineral composition of feline urethral plugs: 1981–2007.

$H_2PO_4^-$, and hydrogen ions are produced during bone mineralization and excreted in urine. If acidic urine is a risk factor for calcium oxalate urolithiasis, a reasonable question would be why calcium oxalate stones are uncommon in immature cats in which urine normally is acidic. The answer likely is related to a combination of risk factors associated with calcium oxalate urolithiasis, including the urine concentrations of minerals, nonmineral crystallization inhibitors and promoters, and the quantity of urine produced, in addition to acid-base balance. There likely is not a simple cause-and-effect relationship between risk factors (eg, urine pH) and calcium oxalate urolithiasis.

Why the prevalence of feline calcium oxalate uroliths are increased, while the prevalence of calcium oxalate in feline urethral plugs remained extremely low (see **Tables 1, 3,** and **5**), is not obvious. This is especially true in light of the observation that male cats tend to be at higher risk for calcium oxalate uroliths and struvite urethral plugs than females. However, the very high prevalence of struvite in urethral plugs is of clinical significance in terms of dietary strategies designed to prevent their formation. The frequency of urethral obstruction of male cats with struvite plugs appears to have

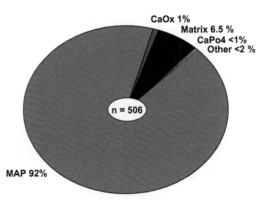

CaOx 1%
Matrix 6.5 %
CaPo4 <1%
Other <2 %

n = 506

MAP 92%

Fig. 9. Mineral composition of feline urethral plugs 2007.

Table 5
Mineral composition[a] of 6,310 domestic feline urethral plugs evaluated at the MUC from 1981 to 2007

Predominant Mineral Type	Number	%
Struvite	5266	83.5
Magnesium hydrogen phosphate	48	0.8
Calcium oxalate	59	0.9
Calcium phosphate	37	0.6
Purines	8	0.1
Magnesium calcium phosphate carbonate	1	<0.1
Mixed[b]	154	2.4
Compound[c]	7	0.1
Matrix	727	11.5
Drug metabolite	1	0.0
Other	2	0.0
Total	6310	100

[a] Analyzed by polarizing light microscopy or infrared spectroscopy.
[b] Urethral plugs did not contain at least 70% of mineral type listed; no nucleus or shell detected.
[c] Urethral plugs contained an identifiable nucleus and one or more surrounding layers of a different mineral type.

been declining during the past two decades. This decline, in all probability, resulted from widespread use of magnesium-restricted or acidifying diets. During the same time period, there has been a dramatic decline in the frequency with which perineal urethrostomies have been performed, and an associated decline in the undesirable sequela of perineal urethrostomies.[7]

A VIEW THROUGH THE RETROSPECTOSCOPE

In the early 1970s, the association between dry diets and feline lower urinary tract disease (LUTD) became a topic of intense discussion in England, Denmark, and the United States.[8] Also in the early 1970s, and continuing sporadically for the next decade, several groups of investigators induced magnesium hydrogen phosphate

Table 6
Mineral composition[a] for 506 feline urethral plugs analyzed at the MUC, 2007

Predominant Mineral Type	Number of Urethral Plugs	%
Magnesium ammonium phosphate $6H_2O$	463	91.5
Magnesium hydrogen phosphate $3H_2O$	2	0.4
Calcium oxalate	5	1.0
Calcium phosphate	2	0.4
Mixed[b]	1	0.2
Matrix	33	6.5
Total	506	100

[a] Analyzed by polarizing light microscopy or infrared spectroscopy.
[b] Urethral plugs did not contain at least 70% of mineral type listed; no nucleus or shell detected.

and then magnesium ammonium phosphate (struvite) uroliths in clinically normal cats by adding various types of minerals to their diets.[8,9,10,11] The cats developed typical signs of LUTD, including urethral obstruction; however, they did not produce the struvite-matrix urethral plugs commonly encountered in cats with naturally occurring urethral obstruction (see **Figs. 10–13**). However, the general consensus of many investigators and clinicians was that consumption of dry diets with excessive magnesium was an important primary cause of lower urinary tract disease of cats.

Following development of dietary protocols to induce dissolution of naturally occurring struvite uroliths in dogs, in 1983, the authors developed dietary protocols to dissolve naturally occurring sterile struvite urocystoliths in cats.[12] Their effectiveness justified further clinical studies on development, detection, dissolution, and prevention of sterile struvite uroliths.

In 1985, results of studies of the effects of feeding diets containing alkalinizing and acidifying salts of magnesium to clinically normal cats were reported.[13] These laboratory studies of induced uroliths shifted the focus of attention from dietary magnesium content to alkaline urine pH as a primary factor in development of struvite crystalluria. These studies had a profound effect on veterinarians and the pet food industry. Many adult feline maintenance diets eventually were modified to minimize struvite crystalluria. Because of dietary modifications, the prevalence of struvite uroliths and struvite urethral plugs began to decline in the mid-1980s, and unexpectedly, the occurrence of calcium oxalate began to increase.

THE CONTINUED PRESENCE OF CALCIUM OXALATE

The exact etiologic cascade of risk factors which lead to the increased prevalence of canine and feline CaOx uroliths remains unknown. However, results of epidemiologic studies support the hypothesis that diets designed to minimize MAP urolith formation may have inadvertently increased the occurrence of CaOx uroliths (see **Figs. 1, 4** and **7**). Several biologic phenomena provide plausible explanations for this association. (1) Whereas diet-mediated urine acidification enhances the solubility of MAP crystals in urine, dietary acids promote calcium oxalate crystalluria by inducing hypercalciuria.[8] This association between aciduria, acidemia, and hypercalciuria may be explained by the fact that acidemia promotes mobilization of carbonate and phosphate from bone to buffer hydrogen ions. Concomitant mobilization of bone calcium may result in hypercalciuria. (2) Metabolic acidosis in dogs, human beings, and rats resulted in hypocitraturia. If consumption of dietary acid precursors is associated with hypocitraturia in cats, it may increase the risk of CaOx uroliths because citrate is an inhibitor of CaOx crystal

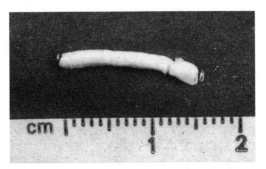

Fig. 10. Feline urethral plug composed of struvite crystals and a large quantity of matrix. (Compare with **Fig. 11.**)

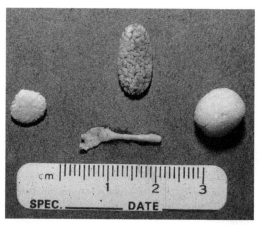

Fig. 11. Sterile struvite urethral plug removed from an adult male cat with urethral obstruction (6 o'clock position). One end of the plug has been crushed with an index finger to illustrate its friable nature. (Compare with **Fig. 10.**) Two wafer-shaped sterile struvite uroliths retrieved from adult male cats are at 9 and 12 o'clock positions. A urocystolith associated with a urease positive urinary tract infection is positioned at the 3 o'clock position.

formation. (3) The widespread practice of feeding low moisture (dry) diets to companion animals resulted in the formation of concentrated urine.

THE AGE OF NEPHROURETEROLITHIASIS

The increase in occurrence of CaOx uroliths in cats has been associated with a parallel increase in occurrence of CaOx uroliths found in their kidneys and ureters (**Figs. 14 and 15**). In fact, there has been a 10-fold increase in the frequency of upper tract uroliths diagnosed in cats evaluated at veterinary teaching hospitals in North America during the past 20 years.[14] Between 1981 and 2003, the MUC analyzed nephroureteroliths retrieved from 2,445 cats: 70% had uroliths composed of calcium oxalate. By contrast, only 8% were composed of MAP (see **Fig. 14**). This finding emphasizes the importance of CaOx prevention and control in cats to minimize potential

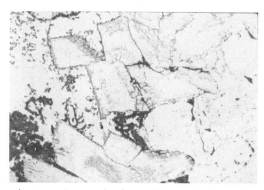

Fig. 12. Transmission electron micrograph of a sterile struvite stone illustrating a paucity of matrix. The clear spaces are areas where the crystals were located. Compare with **Fig. 13.**

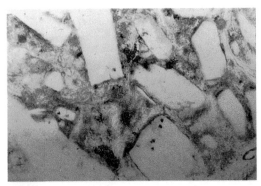

Fig. 13. Transmission electron micrograph of a matrix-crystalline struvite urethral plug retrieved from a cat. Notice the difference in the quantity of matrix between this plug and the stone described in **Fig. 12**.

life-threatening renal failure. The authors are unaware of a parallel increase in calcium oxalate nephroureteroliths in dogs.

Is there an etiologic link between kidney disease and calcium oxalate uroliths? Is kidney disease a cause or consequence of urolith formation? Hyperoxaluria may be the common link between these two processes. One group of investigators reported that excessive oxalic acid damages kidney tubules.[15,16] It is also probable that high concentrations of urine oxalate would be a significant risk factor for the formation of calcium oxalate uroliths in cats. If these assumptions are correct, what is the source of oxalic acid? The answer to these questions likely can be found in the evaluations of various diets.

EPIDEMIOLOGY OF UROLITHIASIS IN HUMAN BEINGS

At the beginning of the twentieth century, the incidence of calcium oxalate uroliths in human beings living in the United States had also dramatically increased.[17] Global distributions of urolithiasis in human beings indicate that calcium oxalate urolithiasis predominates in the United States and other industrialized, technologically advanced

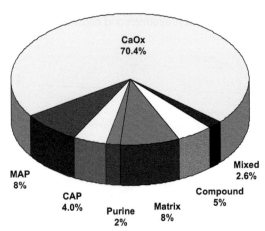

Fig. 14. Prevalence of the mineral types of 2,445 feline nephroureteroliths submitted to the Minnesota Urolith Center for analysis: 1981 to 2007.

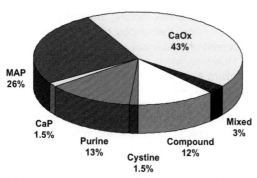

Fig. 15. Prevalence of the mineral types of 5,591 canine nephroureteroliths submitted to the Minnesota Urolith Center for quantitative analysis: 1981 to 2007.

regions of the world. Although originally attributed to the sedentary lifestyle of inhabitants of such countries,[18] the increased incidence of calcium oxalate uroliths now is believed to reflect the ability of these more affluent societies to spend disposable income for the consumption of animal protein, which leads to increased urinary excretion of calcium and oxalate.[11,19] Regional environmental factors, such as water and soil quality, also may influence urolith formation. Because of the close relationship between human beings and their pets, it is logical to consider that risk factors contributing to the increased incidence of calcium oxalate uroliths in human beings also may influence the incidence of calcium oxalate uroliths in cats and dogs. Investigators need to explore the associations between strategies designed to improve nutrition and factors that increase over-nutrition and their relationship to formation of calcium oxalate uroliths.

RISK AND PROTECTIVE FACTORS

The reasons underlying such a dramatic change in the composition of canine and feline uroliths remains a topic of intense interest. Although several hypotheses have been proposed to explain this phenomenon, a cause-and-effect relationship has not yet been established. Not all risk and protective factors are of equal importance. In fact, each contributing risk or protective factor may play a limited or a significant role in the pathogenesis of different types of urolithiasis. The chance of developing a specific type of urolith when exposed to one or more risk or protective factors is often expressed in terms of numerical probabilities (so-called "odds" or "odds ratios").

When used in a qualitative (rather than quantitative) way, the significance of risk or protective factors should not be assigned an "all or none" or "always or never" interpretation.[20] In many situations, each risk factor alone contributes a limited role to the development of urolithiasis. In fact, in some situations, they may not play a role in every exposed patient. Furthermore, identifying one event in a chain of etiologic events is not the same as identifying the entire etiologic chain.

It is apparent that naturally occurring uroliths are affected by many risk factors, some of which are known and some of which are unknown. Some risk factors that influence urolith formation include breed, gender, age, anatomic and functional abnormalities of the urinary tract, abnormalities of metabolism, urinary tract infections, diet, urine pH, and body water homeostasis.

WHY IDENTIFY RISK AND PROTECTIVE FACTORS?

Our interest in recognizing the association of specific risk factors with urolithiasis is related to: 1) identifying healthy but susceptible populations of animals and trying to minimize their exposure to these risk factors; 2) identifying healthy but susceptible populations and trying to enhance their exposure to protective factors; and 3) facilitating detection and treatment of subclinical urolithiasis that has already developed in susceptible patients. However, when several risk factors occur together, they may combine to put the patient at a higher risk than would be expected by the sum of each factor identified (eg, $1 + 1, + 1 = 5$). Recognition and control of lithogenic risk factors is the primary goal to prevent urolith formation and minimize their recurrence.

Because of the short time-span in which the change in the occurrence of mineral types of canine and feline uroliths has been recognized, breed, gender, and age are unlikely to have contributed substantially to this phenomenon. It is the authors interpretation that changes in husbandry and nutrition represent significant contributing factors influencing this epidemiologic shift in urolith type.

FUTURE TRENDS: 10 PREDICTIONS DERIVED VIA THE CRYSTALLURIA BALL

What will be the trends associated with urolithiasis in the future? The authors predict the following advancements in the diagnosis, treatment, and prevention of various types of uroliths during the next decade.

- Our understanding of the pathophysiology of calcium oxalate, sterile struvite, purine, cystine, silica, and calcium phosphate urolithiasis will expand. Their will be new insights into identification of genetic and acquired risk factors associated with this disorder, such that urolithiasis will be further divided into etiopathogenic subsets.
- As techniques of preserving stone matrix are developed, the composition of matrix contained in different mineral types of uroliths will bring additional insights into stone formation.
- Advances will be made in recognition and detection of urolith inhibitors and promoters found in urine. These advances will have diagnostic and therapeutic implications.
- The role of various dietary constituents in the cause and treatment of urolithiasis will be further clarified, based on evidence derived from masked and controlled clinical trials.
- Improvements in the resolution of imagining techniques (such as ultrasonography), and increased familiarity with their use, will allow detection and localization of all types of uroliths less than one millimeter in size.
- Improvements will continue to be made in diagnostic imaging, facilitating identification of the mineral composition of uroliths in vivo.
- Significant advances will be made toward identification of specific diagnostic markers of different types of uroliths in the urine of patients with urolithiasis.
- There will continue to be a decline in the use of invasive therapeutic techniques, such as nephrectomies, nephrotomies, ureterotomies, urocystolithotomies, and urethrotomies. As the pathogenesis of different urolith types are discovered, and as molecular diagnostic strategies are developed and validated, early detection of uroliths will increase the development of medical dissolution and prevention strategies for all urolith types, including calcium oxalate.
- Therapeutic use of minimally invasive types of therapy, such as lithotripsy, will become a standard of practice.
- Veterinary medicine will lead the way in providing information about the causes, detection, and treatment of urolithiasis in animals that is of comparative value to human beings with various types urolithiasis.

REFERENCES

1. Kirk CA, Ling GV, Franti CE, et al. Evaluation of factors associated with development of calcium oxalate urolithiasis in cats. J Am Med Assoc 1995;207:1429–34.
2. Lekcharoensuk C, Osborne CA, Lulich JP, et al. Association between dietary factors and calcium oxalate and magnesium ammonium phosphate uroliths in cats. J Am Vet Med Assoc 2001;219:1228–37.
3. Osborne CA, Kruger JM, Lulich JP, et al. Medical dissolution of feline struvite urocystolithiasis. J Am Vet Med Assoc 1990;196:1053–63.
4. Osborne CA, Kruger JM, Lulich JP, et al. Feline matrix-crystalline urethral plugs: a unifying hypothesis of causes. J Small Anim Pract 1992;33:172–777.
5. Osborne CA, Lulich JP, Thumchai R, et al. Changing demographics of feline urolithiasis. In: August JR, editor. Consultations in feline internal medicine. 3rd edition. Philadelphia: WB Saunders; 1997. p. 349–60.
6. Buffington CAT. Effects of age and food deprivation on urine pH in the cat. In: Proceedings of the 3rd Annual Symposium European Society Veterinary Nephrology Urology 1988. p. 113–21.
7. Lekcharoensuk C, Osborne CA, Lulich JP. Evaluation of trends in frequency of urethrostomy for treatment of urethral obstruction in cats. JAVMA 2002;221:502–5.
8. Osborne CA, Kruger JM, Lulich JP, et al. Feline urologic syndrome; feline lower urinary tract disease; feline interstitial cystitis: what's in a name? J Am Vet Med Assoc 1999;214(10):1470–80.
9. Finco DR, Barsanti JA, Crowell WA. Characterization of magnesium-induced urinary disease in the cat and comparison with feline urologic syndrome. Am J Vet Res 1985;46:391–400.
10. Lewis LD, Chow FHC, Taton GF, et al. Effects of various dietary mineral concentrations on the occurrence of feline urolithiasis. J Am Vet Med Assoc 1978;172:559–63.
11. Rich LJ, Dysart I, Chow FC, et al. Urethral obstruction in male cats: experimental production by addition of magnesium and phosphate to the diet. Feline Pract 1974;4:44–7.
12. Osborne CA, Abdullahi S, Polzin DJ. Current status of dissolution of canine and feline uroliths. In: Proceedings of the Kal Kan Symposium for treatment of small animal diseases. 1983. p. 53–79.
13. Buffington CA, Rogers QR, Morris JG, et al. Feline struvite urolithiasis: magnesium effect depends on urinary pH. Feline Pract 1985;15:29–33.
14. Lekcharoensuk C, Osborne CA, Lulich JP, et al. Evaluation of the trends in the frequency of calcium oxalate uroliths n the upper urinary tract of cats. J Am Anim Hosp Assoc 2005;41:39–46.
15. Robertson WG, Peacock M, Hodgkinson A. Dietary changes and the incidence of urinary calculi in the UK between 1958 and 1976. J Chronic Dis 1979;32:469–76.
16. Turan T, Tuncay OL, Usubutun A, et al. Renal tubular apoptosis after complete urethral obstruction in the presence of hyperoxaluria. Urol Res 2000;28:220–2.
17. Lonsdale K. Human stones. Science 1968;159:199–207.
18. Mandel NS, Mandel GS. Urinary tract stone disease in the United States veteran population II. Geographical analysis of variations in composition. J Urol 1989;1432:11516–21.
19. Robertson WG, Peacock M, Heyburn PJ. Should recurrent calcium oxalate stone formers become vegetarians? Br J Urol 1979;51:427–31.
20. Osborne CA, Lulich JP. Risk and protective factors for urolithiasis. What do they mean? Vet Clin North Am Small Anim Pract 1999;29(1):39–41.

Index

Note: Page numbers of article titles are in **boldface** type.

Vet Clin Small Anim 39 (2008) 199–214
doi:10.1016/S0195-5616(08)00207-6
0195-5616/08/$ – see front matter © 2008 Elsevier Inc. All rights reserved.

vetsmall.theclinics.com

Our issues help you manage *yours.*

Every year brings you new clinical challenges.

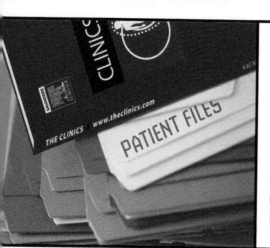

Every **Clinics** issue brings you **today's best thinking** on the challenges you face.

Whether you purchase these issues individually, or order an annual subscription (which includes searchable access to past issues online), the **Clinics** offer you an efficient way to update your know how…one issue at a time.

DISCOVER THE CLINICS IN YOUR SPECIALTY!

Veterinary Clinics of North America: Equine Practice.
Publishes three times a year.
ISSN 0749-0739.

Veterinary Clinics of North America: Exotic Animal Practice.
Publishes three times a year.
ISSN 1094-9194.

Veterinary Clinics of North America: Food Animal Practice.
Publishes three times a year.
ISSN 0749-0720.

Veterinary Clinics of North America: Small Animal Practice.
Publishes bimonthly.
ISSN 0195-5616.

M022483

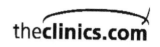

theclinics.com

Moving?

Make sure your subscription moves with you!

To notify us of your new address, find your **Clinics Account Number** (located on your mailing label above your name), and contact customer service at:

E-mail: elspcs@elsevier.com

800-654-2452 (subscribers in the U.S. & Canada)
314-453-7041 (subscribers outside of the U.S. & Canada)

Fax number: 314-523-5170

Elsevier Periodicals Customer Service
11830 Westline Industrial Drive
St. Louis, MO 63146

*To ensure uninterrupted delivery of your subscription, please notify us at least 4 weeks in advance of move.

Printed and bound by CPI Group (UK) Ltd, Croydon, CR0 4YY

03/10/2024

01040463-0002